Gestational Diabetes Mellitus - New Developments

Edited by Miroslav Radenković

Published in London, United Kingdom

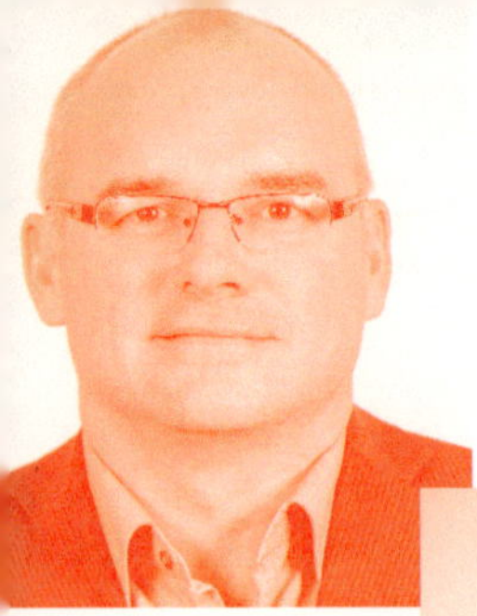
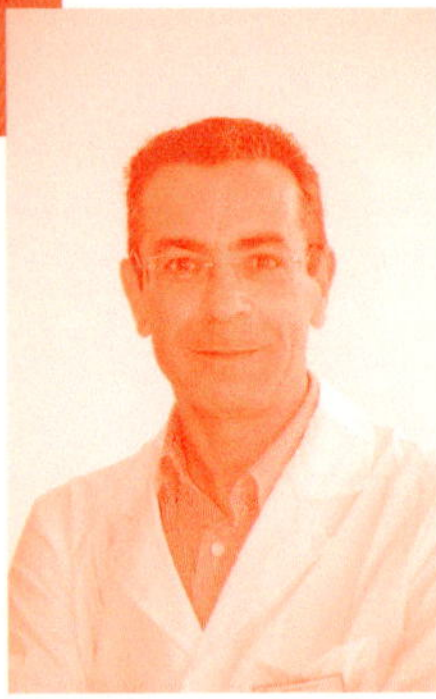
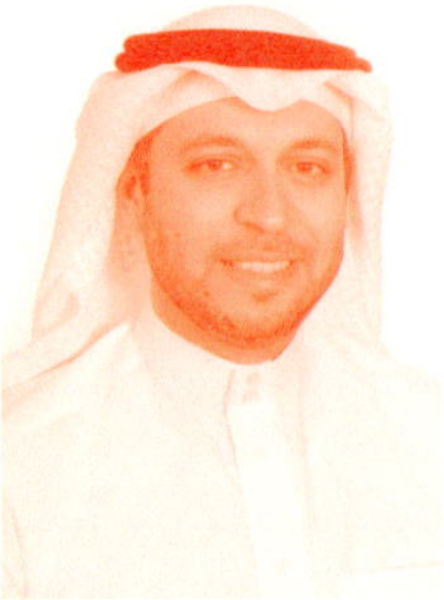
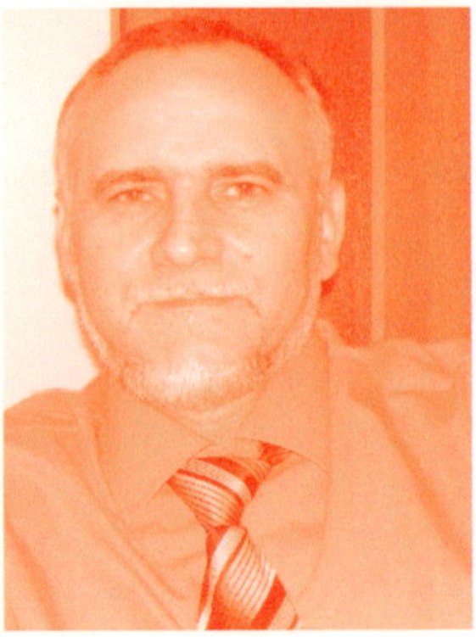
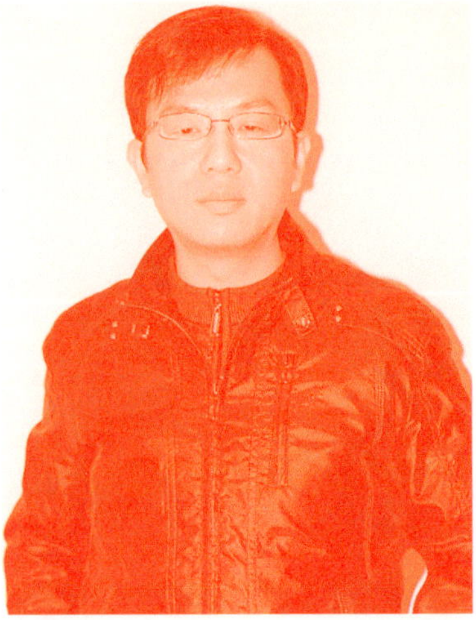
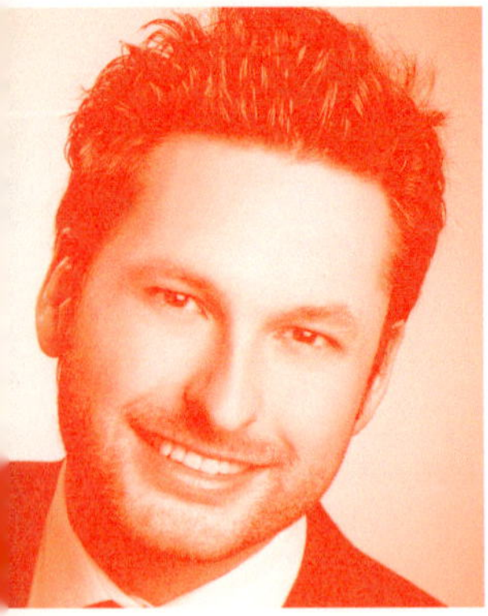
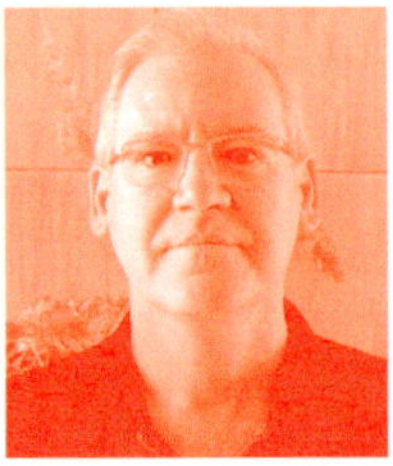

IntechOpen

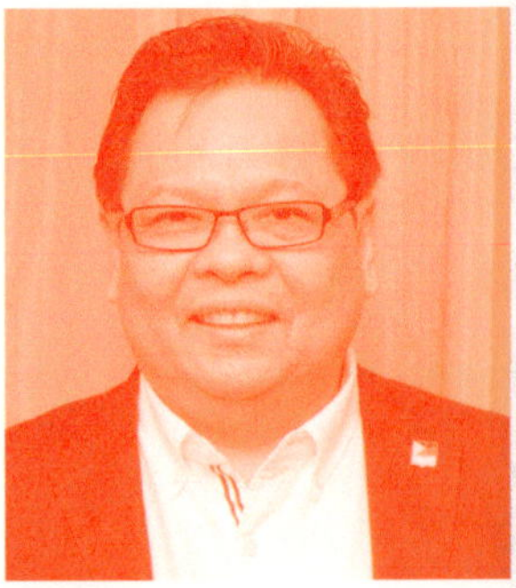
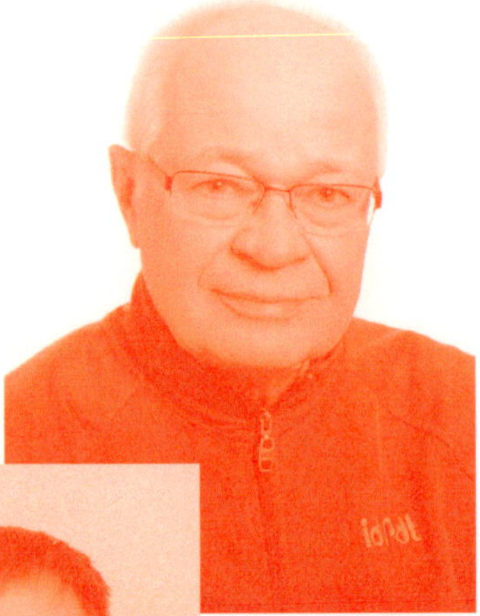
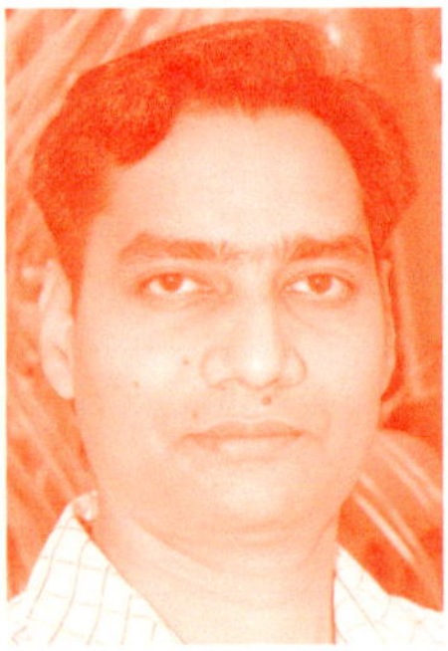
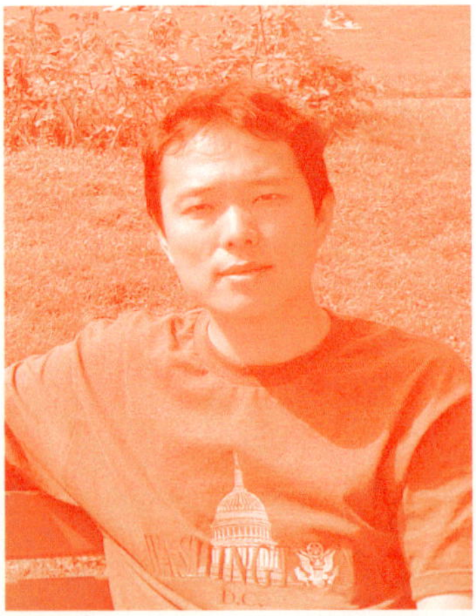
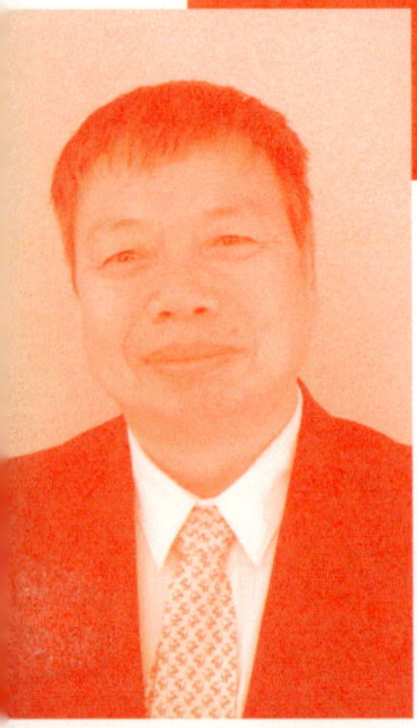
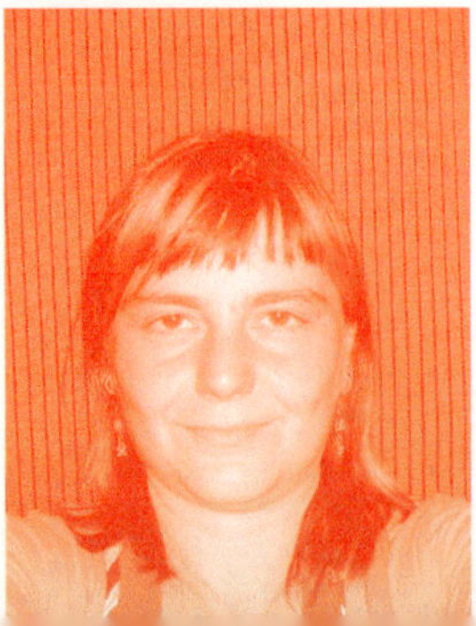

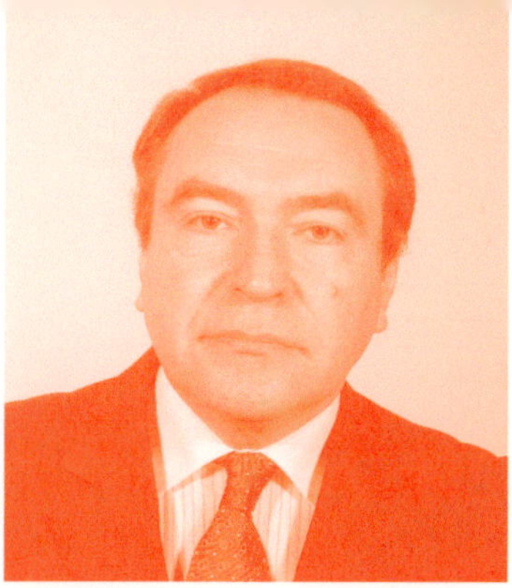
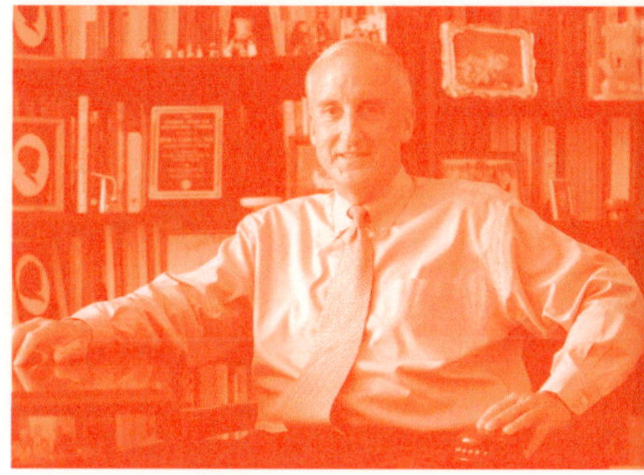
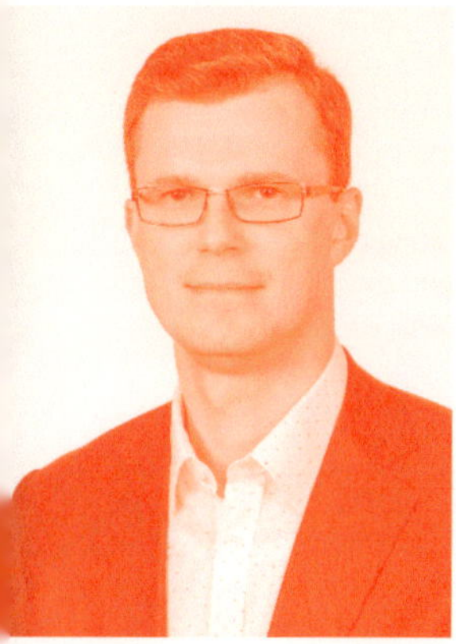
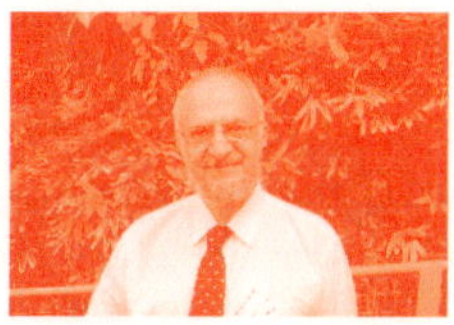
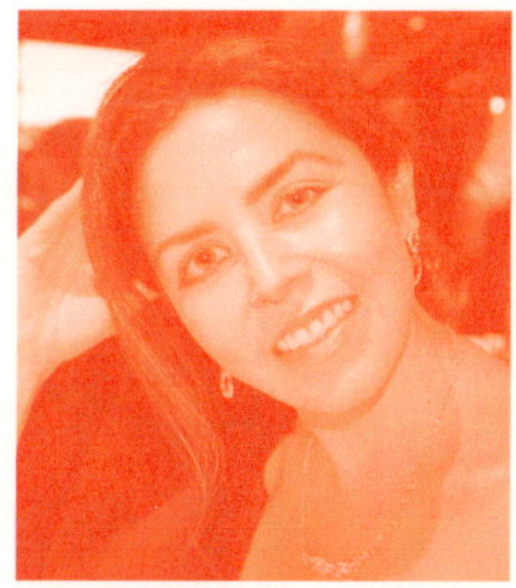

Supporting open minds since 2005

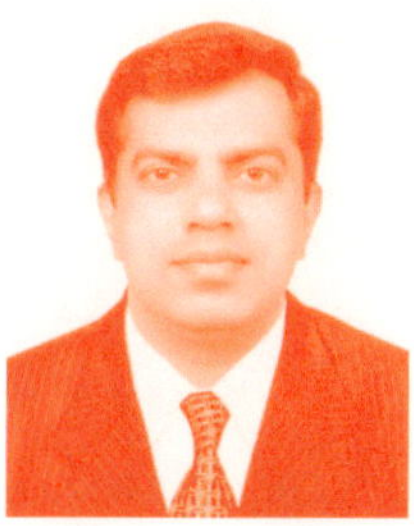
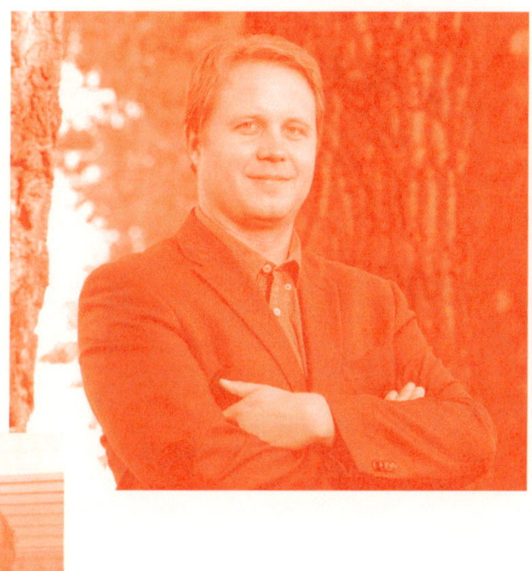
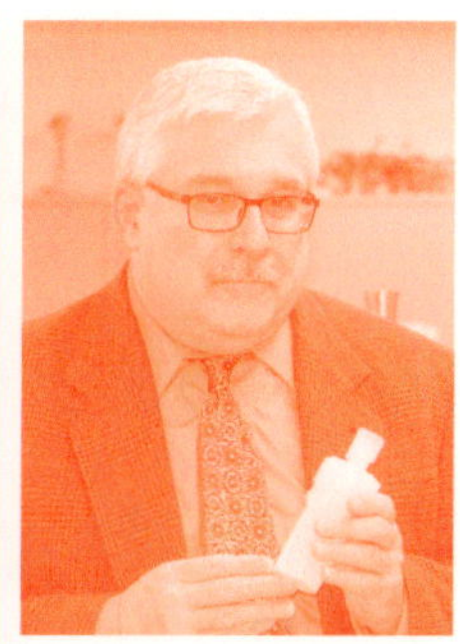
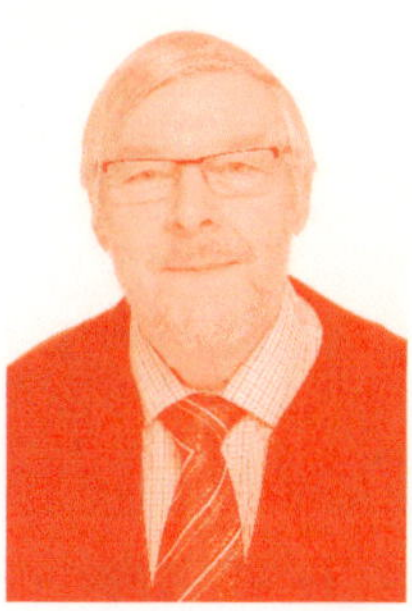
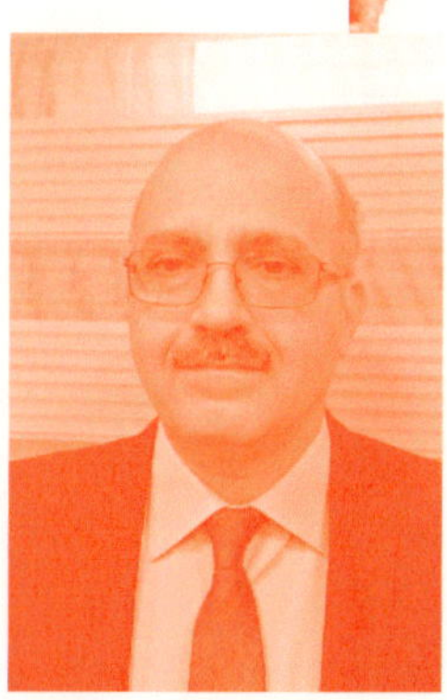
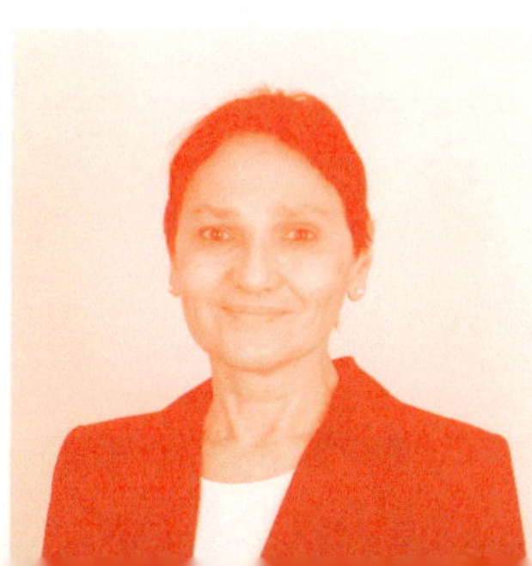
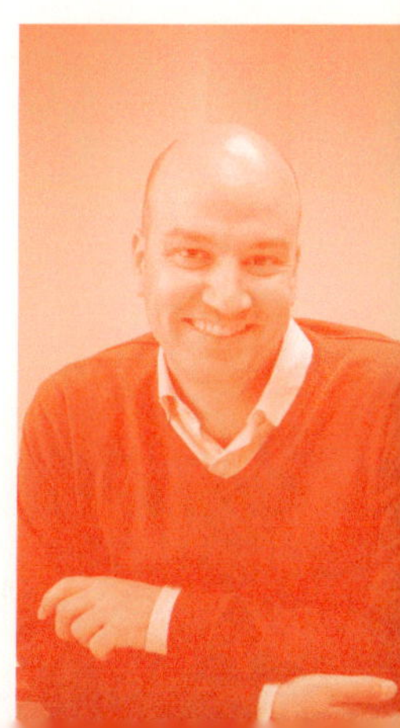

Gestational Diabetes Mellitus - New Developments
http://dx.doi.org/10.5772/intechopen.94687
Edited by Miroslav Radenković

Contributors
Temitope Sanusi-Olubowale, Cristian Espinoza, Dalia Rafat, Samar Banerjee, Akio Nakamura, Ritsuko Kawaharada, Miroslav Radenković, Ana Jakovljević, Brittany R. Allman, Elisabet Børsheim, Samantha McDonald, Linda May, Amber W. Kinsey, Annunziata Lapolla, Silvia Burlina, Maria Grazia Dalfrà, Radiana Staynova, Vesselina Yanachkova

First published in London, United Kingdom, 2022 by IntechOpen
IntechOpen is the global imprint of INTECHOPEN LIMITED, registered in England and Wales, registration number: 11086078, 5 Princes Gate Court, London, SW7 2QJ, United Kingdom
Printed in Croatia

British Library Cataloguing-in-Publication Data
A catalogue record for this book is available from the British Library

Additional hard and PDF copies can be obtained from orders@intechopen.com

Gestational Diabetes Mellitus - New Developments
Edited by Miroslav Radenković
p. cm.
Print ISBN 978-1-83969-818-7
Online ISBN 978-1-83969-819-4
eBook (PDF) ISBN 978-1-83969-820-0

For EU product safety concerns:
IN TECH d.o.o., Prolaz Marije Krucifikse Kozulić 3, 51000 Rijeka, Croatia, info@intechopen.com or visit our website at intechopen.com.

Meet the editor

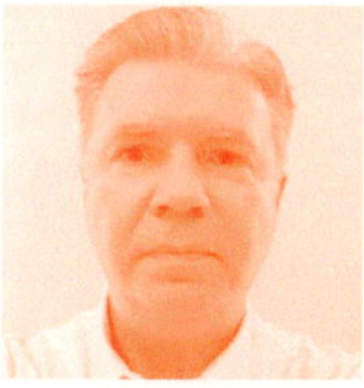

Miroslav Radenković, MD, graduated from the Faculty of Medicine, University of Belgrade (FMUB), Serbia, in 1995, where he also obtained an MS in Pharmacology, board certification in Clinical Pharmacology, a Ph.D. in Medical Sciences, and sub-specialization in Pharmacotherapy in 1999, 2000, 2004, and 2016, respectively. He has worked in the Department of Pharmacology at FMUB since 1996. Dr. Radenković also obtained an MS in Bioethics from Clarkson University, NYC, USA, in 2021. He has participated in several scientific projects supported by the Ministry of Science, Serbia; the Austrian Science Fund; and the NIH Fogarty International Center Project, USA. Dr. Radenković is a member of the Ethics Committee of Serbia.

Contents

Preface

Gestational diabetes mellitus is defined as diabetes diagnosed in the second or third trimester of pregnancy, with no evidence of pre-existing type 1 or type 2 diabetes. Although gestational diabetes normally disappears after delivery, this pathological condition may have long-term medical consequences for both mother and offspring. In accordance, increased risk of miscarriage, macrosomia, complications around delivery, and stillbirth have been clearly connected with diabetes developed during pregnancy.

Although much knowledge has been acquired regarding the prevention, diagnosis, implications, and management of gestational diabetes mellitus, the exact mechanisms of its development are still under investigation. In that way, we can recognize recent efforts in a deeper understanding of the adverse genetic background and the epigenetic modifications linked to nutritional and environmental factors in affecting hyperglycemia of pregnant women and future fetal metabolism.

Pharmacological and non-pharmacological treatments of gestational diabetes are aimed at maintaining euglycemia with regular glucose monitoring, dietary modifications, lifestyle changes, exercise, and appropriate pharmacotherapy.

This book provides a comprehensive overview of recent advances in gestational diabetes mellitus. It includes three major sections directing the reader's attention to the etiology, management, and consequences of the disorder. Chapters present the latest information regarding biomarkers and their promising role in early detection and prevention of gestational diabetes mellitus as well as up-to-date knowledge linked to genetic and epigenetic factors, including gut microbiota. Improving gestational diabetes management through patient education, resistance training throughout pregnancy, and the prudent use of drugs leading to the optimal control of glucose level represent the major components of contemporary management of gestational diabetes mellitus. Unfortunately, despite all medical efforts, gestational diabetes is still connected to some major consequences that may affect both mothers and their offspring. Hence, the closing chapters provided pivotal information regarding vascular injury induced by gestational diabetes mellitus and its relationship with fetal metabolic impairment, maternal microbiome alterations, and finally current data about future risks for children born to mothers with gestational diabetes.

This book is a useful resource for both clinicians and basic investigators to further explore and update existing knowledge on diabetes-related to pregnancy.

We express sincere appreciation to all the chapter authors for their enthusiasm and expertise, as well as IntechOpen for their highly professional and unconditional support.

Dr. Miroslav Radenković
Professor,
Faculty of Medicine,
University of Belgrade,
Belgrade, Serbia

Section 1

Ethology of Gestational Diabetes Mellitus

Chapter 1

Biomarkers in GDM, Role in Early Detection and Prevention

Samar Banerjee

Abstract

Gestational Diabetes Mellitus (GDM) happens to be a very frequent and major complication of pregnancy because of higher morbidity and mortality, both for the mother and the baby. After delivery, GDM carries the risk of higher maternal morbidity due to post pregnancy obesity, development of diabetes mellitus, obesity and also cardiovascular diseases in significant number in both the mother and child for future. As per current guidelines, GDM is diagnosed at the end of the second trimester by elevated blood glucose values when, foetal damages by metabolic and epigenetic changes had already started. As a result, treatments cannot be started before the late second or third trimester, when the process of high risk of foetal morbidity and mortality has been set in. If by any method we can predict development of GDM at earliest part of first trimester or even more overjealously, we can predict, before pregnancy, then and then only we can avoid many disasters induced by GDM. With this idea many biomarkers, both clinical and laboratory based like clinical, metabolic, inflammatory and genetic markers etc., related with early pregnancy metabolic alterations have been studied for their potential to help in the prediction of later pregnancy glucose intolerance. Though promises are seen with some biomarker-enhanced risk prediction models for GDM, but lack of external validation and translation into day-to-day clinical applications, cost effectiveness, with which they may be utilized in routine prenatal care has limited their clinical use. But future is very promising and incorporating the biomarkers which precede the onset of hyperglycaemia into a risk prediction model for GDM and may help us for earlier risk assessment, screening, and diagnosis of GDM and also prevention of its both the immediate and remote complications. This review highlights the current knowledge of the understanding of the candidacy and practical utility of these biomarkers for GDM with recommendations for further research.

Keywords: Biomarkers, gestational diabetes mellitus (GDM), macrosomia, foetal abnormalities

1. Introduction

Norman Freinkel once told that "No single period in human development, provides a greater potential (than pregnancy) for long – range 'pay – off' via a relatively short – range period of enlightened metabolic manipulation".

During pregnancy, the body systems of the woman, must support nutrient and oxygen supply for the proper growth and development of the foetus and subsequently during lactation. Inability to adopt the changes in maternal physiology may lead to complications, such as gestational diabetes mellitus (GDM). The

International Association of Diabetes and Pregnancy Study Groups (IADPSG) shows that, GDM may complicate 15–20% pregnancies, and has increased in the last 20 years in all ethnic groups as much as 27% [1].

GDM originates from interplay of factors like specific gene mutations, dysregulation of placental hormones and β-cell injury, favored by advanced age, gynecological alterations and diabetogenic factors. GDM mostly develop after the 2nd trimester of pregnancy, between the 24th and the 28th week of gestation. GDM may precipitate serious and long-term complications for foetal and maternal health, in particular, metabolism and cardiovascular in nature [2].

Currently, in most cases, the diagnosis of Gestational Diabetes Mellitus (GDM) is done around the late phase of second trimester, which may expose the foetus to the hazards of intrauterine metabolic alterations and also epigenetic changes for the period of exposure. Many documented evidences indicate that the metabolic alterations may subject the new born vulnerable to many long-term pathologies. Detection and management of GDM in pregnancy, can reduce the frequency of adverse pregnancy outcome. Hence, we need to predict and identify GDM earlier in pregnancy even if possible before the pregnancy, in order to limit the exposure to impaired glucose metabolism.

American Diabetes Association (ADA) recommends initial screening for GDM at 24–28 weeks [3]. But Seshiah V et al. from India has detected 62.1% cases of GDM before 24 weeks. Moreover, if we do not test before 24 weeks, we will miss earliest intervention for all the cases of undetected diabetes existing before pregnancy [4].

The aim of this review was to find out the useful and possible markers or guides to detect GDM early in pregnancy before rise of blood sugar and if possible, even before pregnancy to avoid all complication for mother and child arising from effects of GDM on gestation.

1.1 Search strategy and selection criteria

References for this review were identified by searching PubMed, Embase for articles in English with no language restrictions for articles published mainly from 2000 to 2021. The search terms used were GDM biomarkers, GDM pathogenesis, GDM prevention and epigenetics of GDM. The final reference list was prepared based on this search, supplemented with references from the authors' own dataset.

2. Biomarkers

GDM develops when beta cell dysfunction coexists, and is complicated by further abnormalities in adipokine and cytokine profiles, increased free fatty acids (FFA), triglycerides (TG), low vitamin D and endothelial dysfunction. The identification of early biomarkers in pregnancy, who may develop GDM, may lead to an improved understanding of pathogenesis of GDM. Combination of biomarkers and different risk factors into a predictive model, may help in early prediction of GDM. This may also find out effective prevention strategies and finally can limit different complications related with GDM. The first-trimester biochemical predictors of GDM are shown in **Table 1**.

3. Epigenetic footprint

Metabolic alterations like impaired glucose control during the phase of foetal development, may result in functional and structural alterations in the developing foetus, and may result in a predispose to the development of chronic metabolic

- Glycemic markers
  - Fasting glucose
  - Post-load glucose
  - Hemoglobin A1C
  - Serum Insulin
  - Tests of insulin sensitivity (HOMA, QUICKI)
- Lipid profile, with higher concentrations of total cholesterol and triglycerides
- Insulin resistance markers
  - Fasting insulin
  - Sex hormone-binding globulin
- Inflammatory markers
  - C-reactive protein
  - Tumor necrosis factor-alpha
  - IL-6
  - TNF-alfa
  - hsCRP
- Genetic markers rs7957197 (HNF1A), rs10814916 (GLIS3), rs3802177 etc.
- Urine biomarkers: l-tryptophan, l-urobilinogen, ceramide (d18:0/23:0), 21-deoxycortisol, cucurbitacin-C, aspartame etc.
- Adipocyte-derived markers
  - Leptin
  - Adiponectin
  - Resistin
  - Visfatin
  - Omentin-1
  - Ghrelin
- Placenta-derived markers
  - Follistatin-like 3
  - Placental growth factor
  - Placental exosomes
  - afamin,
  - fetuin-A,
  - fibroblast growth factors-21/23,
  - ficolin-3 and follistatin,
  - specific micro- RNAs
- Others
  - Vitamin D
  - Glycosylated fibronectin
  - Soluble(pro)renin receptor
  - Alanine aminotransferase
  - Ferritin
  - Glucagon
  - PAI-1
  - Adipocyte fatty acid-binding protein
  - SNPs,
  - DNA methylation,

Table 1.
Showing the first-trimester biochemical predictors of GDM.

diseases in future life. These alterations are actually the 'foetal programming' and may trigger epigenetic changes [5]. The epigenetic changes are considered as different changes in the biochemical structure of DNA, which alters the gene expression in pregnancy as shown in **Table 2**.

Maternal insulin resistance can also cause insulin resistance in the foetus [6]. Multiple studies have correlated maternal GDM, with the development of obesity and T2DM in children who are eight times more prone to develop T2DM than non-GDM children [7, 8]. This raises the strong need for early detection of GDM preceding the hyperglycaemia which might avoid subsequent harm.

- DNA methylation,
- Histone modification
- Non-coding RNA processes.

Table 2.
Showing the epigenetic changes in pregnancy.

4. Obesity, inflammation and GDM

Now a days, more and more women are becoming pregnant, being either overweight or obese. The obese women show a three-fold risk for developing GDM. The global increase in GDM at present time is largely due to the on-going pandemic of obesity. Obesity is related to an altered production of proinflammatory cytokines from the adipocytes, which may lead to a state of chronic low-grade inflammation. It acts upon the expression and production of different proinflammatory cytokines e.g., TNF-alpha and IL-6 and also many anti-inflammatory cytokines. This also produces adipokines e.g., adiponectin, visfatin and leptin etc. Adipokines can modify insulin secretion & sensitivity, appetite, energy control and inflammation. Sound relationship is evident between obesity, chronic low-grade inflammation and development of T2DM. The normal pregnancy shows a balance between the productions of pro-inflammatory and anti-inflammatory cytokines.

Pregnancies in obese women, further may aggravate the proinflammatory markers and may lead to an imbalance and possible complications. It is now accepted that inflammation is also an associated feature of GDM [9]. During GDM, the increased production of proinflammatory cytokines disturbs the insulin signaling [10]. A down regulation of adiponectin and anti-inflammatory markers such as IL-4 and IL-10 and an enhanced production of proinflammatory cytokines such as IL-6 and TNF-α are usually observed in GDM [11].

5. Adipocyte-derived markers

5.1 Adipokines or Adiponectin's

Adiponectin is actually an adipocyte protein and consists of anti-atherogenic, anti-inflammatory and also insulin-sensitizing effects [12]. Adiponectin is inversely correlated with the clinical conditions like hypertension, dyslipidaemia, obesity and also coronary artery disease. Diminished level of adiponectin are usually seen with an increased risk of T2DM [13]. During the normal pregnancies, adiponectin decrease progressively also, probably from a decrease in insulin sensitivity [14]. Many studies have indicated that reduced adiponectin levels during 24–28 weeks in GDM compared to non GDM women, probably corelate low levels of adiponectin with onset of insulin resistance and diminished beta cell function [15, 16]. In one study, adiponectin concentrations in 560 GDM patients and 781 controls revealed a significantly decreased adiponectin level in GDM patients vs. controls [17].

Adiponectin, an adipokine having anti-inflammatory, anti-atherosclerotic and insulin-sensitizing proprieties in another study, was constantly lower along the 1st–3rd trimester of GDM gestations [18]. Hypoadiponectinemia increases the risk of developing GDM by 4.6 times [19], and is inversely correlated with the insulin resistance, BMI and leptin [20]. The ratio of plasma adiponectin and leptin (< 0.33) is also considered as predictor of GDM as early as the period of 6th to 14th week of pregnancy [21]. But probably the assessment of the high molecular weight oligomeric-adiponectin may give better results [22].

Recent prospective studies have addressed the role of adiponectin as a possible early predictor of GDM. Lower levels of adiponectin in the first trimester of pregnancy are associated with a greater risk for developing GDM. This suggests that a down regulation of adiponectin may be a predictor of GDM [23]. In a systematic review and meta-analysis, adiponectin had a moderate effect for predicting future GDM [24]. Again, a case–control study found revealed that low adiponectin levels in pre-pregnancy period is associated with an increased risk of 5.0-fold for developing GDM [25].

This association was significant even when adjustment of known risk factors for GDM was done. This is important as it can identify a group of high-risk women, who might be not detected by conventional tests. Therapy with adiponectin in animal models of obesity improves glycaemia and also can reduce hyperinsulinaemia without any changes in body weight [26].

To summarize, a lower level of adiponectin is seen with type 2 diabetes, obesity and GDM. Adiponectin may influence the pathophysiology of GDM and also be a promising predictive biomarker for identifying GDM. Subsequent research for lifestyle interventions or adiponectin therapy should be done to finalize the role of adiponectin and diagnostic ability in cases of GDM particularly during the first trimester of GDM. Serum adiponectin in GDM, when is below <8.9 μg/ml shows an odds ratio of 3.3.

5.2 1,5 Alfa anhydroglucitrol, SHBG

Mean value of 1,5 Alfa anhydroglucitrol level is significantly lower in those destined to develop GDM. In the first trimester, higher SHBG levels are indicating the risk of GDM but this was no longer statistically significant when BMI, ethnicity and family history were considered. A measurement of CRP in the first trimester is not a useful marker of GDM [27].

5.3 Leptin

Leptin is an adipocyte-derived hormone, mostly produced by adipocytes but is also produced in ovaries and the placenta. It regulates energy balance through hypothalamic pathways. Increased leptin is associated with weight gain, obesity and hyperinsulinaemia.

Leptin is a proinflammatory adipokine and participate in immune responses. It also affects glucose metabolism by antagonistic action on appetite and insulin action. In addition, it can stimulate oxidative stress, atherogenesis and arterial stiffness [28]. Leptin levels is detected to be significantly higher in the 2nd half of pregnancy in both normal and overweight women with later diagnosis of GDM [29]. Menon M et al. did a prospective observational study with three study groups, with two-time points-first and second trimester to detect gestational diabetes mellitus as follows: [30]

- Normal glucose tolerance (NGT)
- Gestational diabetes mellitus 1 (GDM1), OGCT done at 1st trimester patients diagnosed as GDM in 1st trimester
- Gestational diabetes mellitus 2 (GDM2), Repeat OGCT done at 2nd trimester patients diagnosed as GDM in 2nd trimester.

They found that found that out of the adipokines, leptin was found to be elevated in GDM2 compared to GDM1 and NGT group with a p value (0.11), adiponectin was reduced only in GDM1 group with p value (0.33), TNFα is almost the same in all the 3 study groups but IL-6 is elevated in first and second trimester GDM group.

Maternal leptin levels increase 2 to 3 times in pregnancy, as a placental secretion. Increased levels of leptin have been seen in GDM.

Inflammatory markers like IL-6 and TNF-α also are involved in the pathophysiology of GDM by promoting both the chronic low-grade inflammation and also leptin concentrations. A prospective study detected elevated values of leptin before

16 weeks of conception, regardless of presence of adiposity and this was accompanied by an increased risk of GDM [31]. In another study leptin was increased in all pregnant women, but with highest concentrations in obese GDM patients [32]. But due to confounding effects of the measures of adiposity, current evidence is limited. Leptin is probably involved in the pathophysiology of GDM but is a poor predictor of GDM.

5.4 Visfatin

Visfatin an adipokine mostly secreted from visceral fat. It possesses both endocrine, paracrine and autocrine effects. Increased level of visfatin is noted in obesity, metabolic syndrome and T2DM. During pregnancy, visfatin levels increase up to the 2nd trimester, then they decrease and persist in lowest concentrations in the third trimester. During GDM, studies on visfatin levels are is inconsistent, as both decreased and increased levels have been reported [33].

In addition to its insulin-like properties to bind to the insulin receptor-1 and promotion of hypoglycaemic effects, visfatin can activate NFκB signaling and chemotaxis and lead to the development of insulin resistance. In fact, visfatin was found increased at the late 1st trimester [34], but differentially expressed at the 3rd trimester of GDM [35].

One study observed, visfatin was better in the prediction of GDM in the first trimester than CRP, IL-6, adiponectin and leptin [36]. One case–control study found that, visfatin in the 1st trimester was higher in GDM, but when it was added to the other maternal risk factors, the GDM detection rate had no improvement [37]. At present, findings indicate that visfatin is a potential biomarker for GDM, but we need further prospective studies to further asses the relationship between visfatin and GDM.

5.5 Resistin

Resistin represents an adipose-derived hormone and is expressed from monocytes, macrophages and adipocytes. It is corelated with high LDL-c and pro-inflammatory molecules and is also positively associated with adiposity. It increases during pregnancy, probably from weight gain. A potential link might exist between resistin, adiposity and insulin resistance during pregnancy, but till now, remains inconclusive as because of conflicting reports from case–control studies [38]. Resistin, is found to be reduced or unchanged during GDM [39, 40].

But, nested case–control studies, investigating resistin levels in early pregnancy, found no differences in resistin levels between GDM and controls (adjusted for BMI) [41]. Currently, there is no solid evidence that resistin is involved in the pathophysiology or prediction of GDM.

5.6 Omentin

Omentin-1, is an adipokine produced in non-fat cells from the adipose tissues (stromal vascular cells). It is involved in vascular tone relaxation due to the production of endothelial nitric oxide and lowering of both hs-CRP and TNFα signaling [42]. Omentin-1 was lower at the 2nd trimester of GDM similar to adiponectin, and in contrast to IL-6 [43].

5.7 Ghrelin

Hungarian study reported that fasting serum ghrelin levels were lower in women with GDM compared to non-pregnant healthy controls and pregnant controls without GDM in the 1st trimester and 3rd trimester [44].

6. Inflammatory markers

6.1 TNFα

TNFα a proinflammatory cytokine produced by monocytes and macrophages affects insulin sensitivity and secretion. These occurs from impairment of B-cell function and insulin signaling and results in insulin resistance and possibly GDM [45]. Multiple studies showed increased maternal TNFα levels in GDM, predominantly during late pregnancy [46]. Increased TNF-α levels in GDM than controls have been shown. Subgroup analysis detected this relationship to remain significant when they are compared with BMI-matched controls [47].

These increased levels are due to increased oxidative stress and inflammation arising from impaired glucose metabolism [48]. A small case–control study Of 14 cases and 14 controls to address the predictive value of TNFα found no differences between women with GDM and without [49]. In one study of GDM and controls, TNFα levels measured pre-gravid, at 12–14 weeks and 34–36 weeks were increased at 34–36 weeks of gestation. These were inversely correlated with the insulin sensitivity [50]. We need more prospective studies to assess the predictive value of TNFα during GDM, with due adjustment for measures of adiposity.

6.2 Il-6

IL-6 is one of the proinflammatory cytokines and is increased in obesity and associated with indices of adiposity and insulin resistance, such as body mass index (BMI). The relationship between IL-6 and insulin action appears to be regulated via adiposity. However, in a case–control study, plasma IL-6 levels were elevated when adjusted for BMI in women with GDM [51].

6.3 High-sensitivity C-reactive protein (hsCRP)

Wolf and co-workers had found that the first-trimester CRP levels were significantly raised among them who later on developed GDM than the control subjects (3.1 vs. 2.1 mg/L, $P < 0.01$) [52]. After the adjustment for age, race/ethnicity, blood pressure smoking, parity, and age at gestation at CRP sampling, the increased risk of developing GDM among women was seen in the highest tertile than the lowest tertile and was 3.6 times higher (95% CI: 1.2–11.4). But when adjusted for BMI, this relation was not seen anymore. But Berggren and co-workers examined whether first-trimester hs CRP could predict the third-trimester impaired glucose tolerance (IGT). The hs CRP was positively correlated to (hs)CRP and GDM appears to be partly mediated by BMI.

Another study found that elevated plasma insulin and reduced adiponectin levels during first trimester may improve GDM identification rates than by clinical factors alone [53]. Maternal risk factors alone offer a prediction rate of 61% for GDM, but addition of adiponectin and SHBG, improved detection rates to 74% [54].

7. Glycaemic markers

7.1 Serum insulin and C-peptide

O'Malley E G et al. found that, both the serum insulin and C-peptide levels in the third tertile were correlated with GDM development ($p < 0.001$ if adjusted for maternal obesity). Higher values of ghrelin were showing a lower odd of development of GDM, even after adjustment for maternal obesity. The conclusion of the study was though 3 of the 10 biomarkers were statistically indicating an increased risk of GDM, but the presence of large overlap in values between women with normal and abnormal glucose tolerance reflect that the biomarkers (alone or in combination) were not clinically helpfull [55].

7.2 Glucagon and PAI-1

Two small studies of 54 and 51 women reported higher levels of glucagon and PAI-1 respectively in women with GDM [56, 57].

8. Serum lipids

Li et al. compared 379 women in the first trimester who developed GDM subsequently with 2166 healthy women. They found that lipid profile was different between the groups. The GDM patients had higher concentrations of Triglyceride, LDL-Cholesterol and total cholesterol but lower concentrations of HDL [58]. The lipid values at first trimester in the cohort of Correa et al. was altered even when glycaemia and glycated hemoglobin were normal. The first trimester insulin concentration was seen to be also higher in women who developed GDM. Both theses indicate that there is a role of lipid metabolism in the pathogenesis of the disease [59].

9. Placenta-related factors

Placenta-Related Factors such as sex hormone-binding globulin, afamin, fetuin-A, fibroblast growth factors-21/23, ficolin-3 and follistatin, or specific micro- RNAs may be involved in GDM progression and may help in its recognition [60].

In GDM, some adipose-derived factors such as TNFα, visfatin, omentin and FABP4 may be also expressed and expressed from placenta, resulting to their elevated plasma levels [10]. The sex hormone binding globulin (SHBG) from placenta acting as a regulator of sex steroid hormones had been linked with inversely insulin resistance, metabolic syndrome, obesity and T2DM [61]. A lower level of plasma SHBG in the 1st trimester was a true biomarker for GDM [62, 63].

Nanda et al. showed reduced SHBG in parallel to adiponectin in GDM during 11–13th week of pregnancy, in presence of previous macrosomia, BMI > 30 kg/m2, and family history of DM [63, 64]. Similarly, an hepatokine promoter of insulin resistance, known as fetuin-B, is raised at the 3rd trimester of GDM, but returns after delivery [65]. Again, at the late 1st trimester, a reduction of plasma fetuin-A levels (and elevated hs-CRP) is also noted [66].

FGF-21, responsible for browning of white adipose tissue and an upstream effector of adiponectin, was increased in GDM at the 24th week of gestation [67]. Afamin, a glycoprotein member of the albumin family found in liver and placenta, may be a first trimester biomarker for pathological glucose and lipid metabolism [68].

The decreased levels of ficolin-3 (an activator of the lectin pathway of the complement system expressed in liver and placenta) and the increased ratio of ficolin-3/adiponectin are predictive of GDM at the 16–18th week of gestation [18]. Follistatin, a gonadal regulator of follicular-stimulant hormone and activin-A, having angiogenic, anti-inflammatory and cardioprotective properties, were lower in the 3rd trimester of GDM pregnancy [69].

The non-coding RNAs such as micro-RNAs (miR) can be released from placenta to maternal circulation as early as the 6th week of gestation and may be involved in placenta development, insulin signaling and cardiovascular homeostasis [70]. These miR can regulate trophoblasts proliferation, apoptosis, migration and invasion, and angiogenesis [71].

A significant downregulation of miR-29a, miR-132 and miR-222 had been reported in plasma at the 16th week of pregnant women who developed GDM [72]. Similarly, during the 7th–23rd week of gestation, elevated plasma levels of miR-21-3p were seen with GDM [73].

9.1 Sex hormone-binding globulin (SHBG)

SHBG a glycoprotein regulates the transport of sex hormones. In vitro, this is a marker in insulin resistance as insulin and insulin-like growth factor inhibit SHBG secretion. Indeed, a relation of low levels of SHBG and T2DM has been observed [74]. A study found its concentrations to be significantly lower in GDM [75]. Moreover, women treated with insulin showed even lower SHBG levels. Probably SHBG may help to differentiate or predict who will require insulin therapy or not.

A prospective study evaluated several biomarkers before 15 weeks of gestation and observed that low levels of SHBG were indicating an increased risk of GDM. Adding hs-CRP increases the specificity to 75.46% [76]. However another prospective cross-sectional study, revealed that low levels of SHBG assessed between 13 and 16 weeks of gestation were positively associated with the development of GDM ($n = 30$) ($P < 0.01$) [77]. A case–control study also found that SHBG in the non-fasting state in first trimester had a consistent association with an increased GDM risk [78].

10. Other potential biomarkers

AFABP or Adipocyte fatty acid-binding protein may be one of the risk predictors for cardiovascular disease, metabolic syndrome and T2DM [79]. Two studies have established its increased levels in GDM. Gestational diabetes mellitus causes changes in the concentrations of adipocyte fatty acid-binding protein and other adipo-cytokines in cord blood [80, 81]. Studies investigating the predictive value of AFABP in GDM have not been performed to date, however.

The fatty acid-binding protein 4 (FABP4) correlates with obesity markers e.g., fat mass and high BMI. FABP4 act on lipid and glucose metabolism via fatty acid transport and uptake [82]. The retinol-binding protein 4 (RBP4) is one of the circulating retinol transporters and id correlated with cardiometabolic markers in inflammatory chronic diseases like T2DM, metabolic syndrome obesity, and atherosclerosis process [83]. Higher levels of FABP4 can predict GDM from the 1st and 3rd trimester of [84, 85]. Upregulated values of plasma RBP4 in the 1st and 2nd trimester may modestly indicate GDM risk, especially among women with obesity and advanced age [18, 86].

10.1 Molecular biomarkers

Growing evidence suggests the use of SNPs, DNA methylation, and miRNAs as biomarkers that could help in the early detection of GDM. In presence of their potential, these molecular biomarkers pose several challenges that need to be addressed before they can become clinically applicable [87].

Decreased levels of first trimester pregnancy-associated plasma protein A (PAPP-A) and increased levels of second trimester unconjugated estriol (uE3) and dimeric inhibin A (INH) were associated with GDM [88].

10.2 Vitamin D

Lower levels of vitamin D have been seen in both obesity and type 2 diabetes and also in pregnancy very often. Low levels of Vitamin D levels during first trimester also carry a higher risk for GDM as seen in recent meta-analyses [89]. As the mentioned studies all were not randomized controlled studies, we need future RCTs to confirm the predictive role of vitamin D [90].

10.3 Candidate proteins

Zhao et al. studied maternal blood prospectively from pregnant women at 12–16 weeks of pregnancy. Among these, 30 women were subsequently diagnosed with GDM at 24 to 28 weeks and were selected as case studies along with 30 normoglycemic women as controls. They found that, four proteins, apolipoprotein E, coagulation factor IX, fibrinogen alpha chain, and insulin-like growth factor-binding protein 5, with a high sensitivity and specificity, may provide effective early screening for GDM. The panel of four candidate proteins could distinguish women subsequently developed with GDM from controls with high sensitivity and specificity [91].

10.4 Genetic markers

For the first time, Ding M et al. detected 8 variants to be associated with GDM, They are rs7957197 (HNF1A), rs3802177 (SLC30A8), rs10814916 (GLIS3), rs34872471 (TCF7L2), rs9379084 (RREB1), rs7903146 (TCF7L2), rs11787792 (GPSM1) and also rs7041847 (GLIS3). They also confirmed 3 other variants e.g., rs1387153 (MTNR1B), rs10830963 (MTNR1B), and rs4506565 (TCF7L2), which had been earlier identified by them or significant association with GDM risk [92].

10.5 Urine biomarkers

The study of urine metabolome profile in GDM during the 3rd trimester found relation of 14 metabolites with the steroid hormone biosynthesis and tryptophan metabolism, which were significantly high. They are l-urobilinogen, l-tryptophan, 21-deoxycortisol, cucurbitacin-C, ceramide (d18:0/23:0) and aspartame [93]. Upregulation of these pathways could aggravate insulin resistance and respond to oxidative stress and inflammation during GDM. Earliest at 12th–26th week of pregnancy, augmented levels of AHBA, 3-hydroxybutanoic acid (BHBA), valine, alanine, serotonin and related metabolites like l-tryptophan levels were observed in urine (and plasma) from GDM mothers [94].

11. Clinical prediction models incorporating biomarkers

Clinical risk prediction models' wave has been investigated in GDM. For example, the development of GDM can be predicted from the ethnicity, family history, history of GDM and body mass index. One large prospective study (n = 7929), found that, based on BMI, ethnicity, family history of diabetes and past history of GDM, there was a sensitivity, specificity and AUC of 73% [66–79], 81% [80–82] and 0.824 (0.793–0.855), respectively, for the identification of GDM patients who required insulin therapy [95].

The introduction of biomarkers if added to a set of clinical risk factors are supposed to increase the predication rates of GDM. In particular, low HDL cholesterol and tissue plasminogen activator (t-PA) appeared as independent significant predictors of GDM. The addition of these 2 biomarkers to a group of clinical and demographic risk factors enhances the ROC (area under the curve) from 0.824 to 0.861 [96]. The t-PA not only is a predictor of GDM, it is also associated with a higher risk of T2DM [97].

Addition of maternal adiponectin and visfatin to a bunch of maternal risk factors, reached a detection rate of 68% [98]. The clinical implementation of these multi-parametric prediction models is determined by factors like practical acceptability, significant reduction in adverse pregnancy outcomes and cost-effectiveness. But these models need prospective validation studies and also further identification of predictive threshold values for the said biomarkers.

12. Metabolomic profiling

In one study, women with GDM (n = 96) were matched to women with NGT (n = 96) by age, BMI, gravidity and parity and the levels of 91 metabolites measured. Six metabolites (anthranilic acid, alanine, glutamate, creatinine, allantoin and serine) were found to have significantly different levels between the two groups in conditional logistic regression analyses ($p < 0.05$). Metabolic markers identified as being predictive of type 2 diabetes may not have the same predictive power for GDM [99].

Endogenous galanin as a novel biomarker to predict gestational diabetes mellitus is also observed [100]. The higher level of galanin observed in GDM may represent an adaptation to the rise of glucose, weight, GGT associated with GDMs thriving for clinically useful thresholds [101].

Mean 1,5 AG levels are significantly lower in those that go on to develop GDM. Hs-CRP and SHBG are important early predictors of GDM. Adding SHBG to hs-CRP improves specificity and serves good overall accuracy. Uric acid, creatinine and albumin have no role in GDM prediction [102].

Bivariate logistic regression analysis had shown that both adiponectin and insulin highlight future development of gestational diabetes. Both of them measured at 11 weeks, may predict oncoming GDM. But we need further studies to assess the reliability of these biomarkers [103].

Placental growth factor (PLGF), a vascular endothelial growth factor-like protein, is highly expressed in the placenta. About three studies suggest that higher early pregnancy PLGF levels are associated with GDM [104–106]. Recently, ALT, a liver enzyme, a marker of hepatocellular damage, has been examined as a first-trimester predictor of GDM [107].

One moderate-sized study (N = 182) showed that glycosylated fibronectin measured in the first trimester could predict GDM with high accuracy [108]. Watanabe et al. assessed the soluble (pro)renin receptor levels in 716 Japanese women at less than 14 weeks of gestation and found increased levels in women who developed subsequent GDM [109]. In a case–control study of 1000 women from the UK, Syngelaki et al. found that maternal serum TNF-alpha measured at 11–13 weeks gestation was associated with subsequent GDM [110].

Donovan et al. in their study, indicated that women diagnosed with GDM have lower first trimester levels of both pregnancies associated free β-hCG and plasma protein-A (PAPP-A) than normoglycemic pregnant women. These two markers may indicate the presence of abnormal glucose metabolism at the beginning of pregnancy and may help for identification of future development of GDM [111].

13. First trimester biomarkers for prediction of gestational diabetes mellitus

Tenenbaum-Gavish et al. in a cohort of GDM group found that, compared to the normal group BMI and insulin (P = 0.003) were higher (both P < 0.003). The soluble (s)CD163 and multiples of median values of uterine artery pulsatility index (UtAPI) were high (p for both <0.01) but, pregnancy associated plasma protein A, tumor-necrosis factor alpha and placental protein 130, were low (p for all <0.005). There was no significant difference between the groups in placental growth factor, leptin, interleukin 6, soluble mannose receptor or peptide YY. For screening GDM in obese pregnancy a combination of high BMI, TNFα, insulin and sCD163 reached an AUC of 0.95, and the detection rate of 89% with a 10% false positive rate. For nonobese pregnancy, the combination of TNFα, PP13,sCD163 and PAPP-A showed an AUC of 0.94 and the detection rate was 83% at 10% false positive rate [112].

14. Conclusion

By blood sugar estimation when GDM is diagnosed, adverse foetal changes have already set in. So, we will have to attempt to diagnose GDM, before the foetal changes take place. It would be more rewarding if we can diagnose impending GDM and alert the person even when she plans for pregnancy.

Different biomarkers e.g., glycemic, insulin resistance, inflammatory, adipocyte and placenta-derived, had been evaluated as the first-trimester predictors of GDM. The majority of these studies are smaller in size and was based on case–control designs. But some large studies of glycemic markers indicated that hemoglobin A1C and/or fasting glucose help in detecting women without diagnosis of previous diabetes and they may be benefited from early detection and treatment of GDM, though these observations should be confirmed by interventional studies.

The improvement of GDM development and outcomes is possible by earlier and more specific identification of GDM accompanied by metabolic and cardiovascular risks. In line with these, first or second trimester-related biomarkers seen in maternal plasma like adipose tissue-derived factors like adiponectin, omentin-1, visfatin, fatty retinol binding-protein-4 and acid-binding protein-4 reflect correlations with development of GDM. In addition, placenta-related factors e.g., sex hormone-binding globulin, afamin, fetuin-A, ficolin-3 and follistatin, fibroblast growth factors-21/23 and specific micro-RNAs may be important in detecting progression of GDM and its recognition. Finally, urinary metabolites related to non-polar amino-acids and ketone bodies, serotonin system, may help in completing a predictive or early diagnostic group of GDM biomarkers.

To transform the observations obtained from observational studies into clinical practice, we need also more clinical trials or cost-effectiveness analyses of screening and treatment c.onsidering the first-trimester biochemical GDM predictors. Further studies should examine the first-trimester biochemical markers for adverse outcomes in GDM by prospective trials to find its prevention or early treatment.

GDM involves a significant proportion of pregnant women and is becoming more prevalent as rates of obesity rise globally. Its development and complications could be arrested if accurately predicted in early pregnancy even if possible before conception and effective interventions initiated. Many Several biomarkers have been studied to understand pathogenesis of GDM, but till date none are showing adequate robustness to be used for clinical algorithms for prediction of GDM.

Application of the high methodologies gives novel insights about the role of genetic variants, metabolomics and epigenetics regarding the pathogenesis of GDM. This option for using a predictive model during the subclinical phase of GDM appears to be promising as an important arena of future research and development. These modern technologies are off course complex and not applicable to mass level screening. There are also issues related to validity across populations, reproducibility, and selectivity. We will have to find out methods with cost-effectiveness and universal access, otherwise the present complex biomarkers are likely to prove invaluable in the diagnosis of GDM.

The emerging evidences suggest that the assessment at eleven and thirteen weeks of gestation, should be the platform towards a new approach in antenatal care. The data from the maternal history should be added to the results of biochemical and biophysical tests to examine the patient-specific risk related to a wide variety of pregnancy complications. Ideal GDM biomarkers appears to be a combination of several molecular biomarkers to balance the lack of sensitivity and specificity of individual factors. But targeted rapid technological advances will overcome these challenges and develop a quick, cost-effective point-of-care test that can accurately identify women at high risk for GDM during early pregnancy even if before conception.

Author details

Samar Banerjee
Department of Medicine and Specialist Diabetes Clinic, Vivekananda Institute of Medical Sciences, Kolkata, India

*Address all correspondence to: drsamarbanerjee@gmail.com

References

[1] Ferrara A. Increasing prevalence of gestational diabetes mellitus: a public health perspective. Diabetes Care. 2007;30: S141–S6.5.

[2] Pedersen J. Diabetes and pregnancy; blood sugar of new born infants during fasting and glucose administration. Ugeskr Laeger.1952;114(21):68.4.

[3] American Diabetes Association. Management of Diabetes in Pregnancy: Standards of Medical Care in Diabetes 2021.Diabetes Care 2021;44(Suppl. 1): S200–S210.

[4] Seshiah V, Cynthia A, Balaji V, Balaji M S, Arthi T. Detection and care of women with gestational diabetes mellitus from early weeks of pregnancy results in birth weight of new born babies appropriate for gestational age. Diabetes research and clinical practice, 2008, vol. 80, 2, pp. 199-202.

[5] Hanson M A and Gluckman P. D. Early Developmental Conditioning Of Later Health And Disease: Physiology Or Pathophysiology? Physiological Reviews 2014 94 1027-1076.).

[6] Cardozo E, Pavone M E,Jennifer E. et al. Metabolic syndrome and oocyte quality. Trends in Endocrinology and Metabolism 2011 22 103-109.

[7] Crume TL, Ogden L, Daniels S et al. The impact of in utero exposure to diabetes on childhood body mass index growth trajectories: the EPOCH study Journal of Pediatrics 2011 158 941-946.

[8] Clausen T D, Mathiesen E R, Hansen T et al. High Prevalence of Type 2 Diabetes and Pre-Diabetes in Adult Offspring of Women with Gestational Diabetes Mellitus or Type 1 Diabetes – The Role of Intrauterine Hyperglycemia. Diabetes Care 2008 31 340-346.

[9] Qiu C, Sorensen TK, Luthy DA et al. A prospective study of maternal serum C-reactive protein (CRP) concentrations and risk of gestational diabetes mellitus. Paediatric and Perinatal Epidemiology 2004 18 377-384

[10] Kirwan J P, Mouzon S H, Lepercq J et al. TNF-α is a predictor of insulin resistance in human pregnancy. Diabetes 2002 51 2207-2213.

[11] Georgiou H M, Lappas M, Georgiou GM et al. Screening for biomarkers predictive of gestational diabetes mellitus. Acta Diabetologica 2008 45 157-165.

[12] Chandran M, Phillips SA, Ciaraldi T et al. Adiponectin: more than just another fat cell hormone? Diabetes Care 2003 26 2442-2450.

[13] Nakashima R, Kamei N, Yamane K al. Decreased Total and High Molecular Weight Adiponectin Are Independent Risk Factors for the Development of Type 2 Diabetes in Japanese-Americans. Americans. Journal of Clinical Endocrinology and Metabolism 2006 91 3873-3877.

[14] Galic S, Oakhill JS, Steinberg GR Adipose tissue as an endocrine organ. Molecular and Cellular Endocrinology 2010 316 129-139.

[15] Tsai PJ, Yu CH, Hsu SP et al Maternal plasma adiponectin concentrations at 24 to 31 weeks of gestation: negative association with gestational diabetes mellitus. Nutrition 2005 21 1095-1099.

[16] Soheilykhah S, Mohammadi M, Mojibian M et al. Maternal serum adiponectin concentration in gestational diabetes. Gynecological Endocrinology 2009 25 593-596.

[17] Xu J, Zhao YH, Chen YP et al. Maternal circulating concentrations of

tumor necrosis factor-alpha, leptin, and adiponectin in gestational diabetes mellitus: a systematic review and meta-analysis. Scientific World Journal 2014 2014 926-932.

[18] Yuan X-S, Shi H, Wang H-Y, Yu B, Jiang J. Ficolin-3/adiponectin ratio for the prediction of gestational diabetes mellitus in pregnant women. J Diabetes Investig. 2018; 9:403-410.

[19] Williams MA, Qiu C, Muy-Rivera M, Vadachkoria S, Song T, Luthy DA. Plasma adiponectin concentrations in early pregnancy and subsequent risk of gestational diabetes mellitus. J Clin Endocrinol Metab. 2004;89:2306-2311.

[20] Cseh K, Baranyi E, Melczer Z, Kaszás E, Palik E, Winkler G. Plasma adiponectin and pregnancy-induced insulin resistance. Diabetes Care.2004; 27:274-275.

[21] Thagaard IN, Krebs L, Holm J-C, Lange T, Larsen T, Christiansen M. Adiponectin and leptin as first trimester markers for gestational diabetes mellitus: a cohort study. Clin Chem Lab Med. 2017;55:1805-1812.

[22] Abell SK, Shorakae S, Harrison CL, Hiam D, Moreno-Asso A, Stepto NK, et al. The association between dysregulated adipocytokines in early pregnancy and development of gestational diabetes. Diabetes Metab Res Rev. 2017;33(8):e2926.

[23] Wójcik M, Chmielewska-Kassassir M, Grzywnowicz K et al. The relationship between adipose tissue-derived hormones and gestational diabetes mellitus (GDM). Endokrynologia Polska 2014 65 134-142.

[24] Iliodromiti S, Sassarini J, Kelsey TW et al. Accuracy of circulating adiponectin for predicting gestational diabetes: a systematic review and meta-analysis. Diabetologia 2016 59 692-699.).

[25] Hedderson M M, Darbinian J, Havel P J et Low Prepregnancy Adiponectin Concentrations Are Associated With a Marked Increase in Risk for Development of Gestational Diabetes Mellitus.al. Diabetes Care 2013 36 3930-3937.

[26] Ukkola O, Santaniemi M. Adiponectin: a link between excess adiposity and associated comorbidities? Journal of Molecular Medicine 2002 80 696-702.

[27] Corcoran SM, Achamallah N, Loughlin JO et al. First trimester serum biomarkers to predict gestational diabetes in a high-risk cohort: Striving for clinically useful thresholds. Eur J Obstet Gynecol Reprod Biol. 2018 Mar; 222: 7-12. Epub 2018 Jan 1.

[28] Katsiki N, Mikhailidis DP, Banach M. Leptin, cardiovascular diseases and type 2 diabetes mellitus. Acta Pharmacol Sin. 2018; 39:1176-1188.

[29] López-Tinoco C, Roca M, Fernández-Deudero A, García-Valero A, Bugatto F, Aguilar-Diosdado M, et al. Cytokine profile, metabolic syndrome and cardiovascular disease risk in women with late-onset gestational diabetes mellitus. Cytokine. 2012; 58:14-19.

[30] Menon M, Alaganandha M, Mohan J et al. Int J Reprod Contracept Obstet Gynecol. 2017 Oct;6(10):4402-4406.

[31] Qiu C, Williams MA, Vadachkoria S. Increased maternal plasma leptin in early pregnancy and risk of gestational diabetes mellitus. Obstetrics & Gynecology 2004 103 519-525.

[32] Kirwan JP, Mouzon S H, Lepercq J et al. TNF-α is a predictor of insulin resistance in human pregnancy. Diabetes 2002 51 2207-2213.

[33] Lewandowski KC, Stojanovic N, Press M et al. Elevated serum levels of

visfatin in gestational diabetes: a comparative study across various degrees of glucose tolerance. Diabetologia 2007 50 1033-1037.

[34] Ferreira AFA, Rezende JC, Vaikousi E, Akolekar R, Nicolaides KH. Maternal serum visfatin at 11-13 weeks of gestation in gestational diabetes mellitus. Clin Chem. 2011; 57:609-613.

[35] Rezvan N, Hosseinzadeh-Attar MJ, Masoudkabir F, Moini A, Janani L, Mazaherioun M. Serum visfatin concentrations in gestational diabetes mellitus and normal pregnancy. Arch Gynecol Obstet. 2012; 285:1257-1262.

[36] Mastorakos G, Valsamakis G, Dimitrios C.et al. The Role of Adipocytokines in Insulin Resistance in Normal Pregnancy: Visfatin Concentrations in Early Pregnancy Predict Insulin Sensitivity. Clinical Chemistry 2007 53 1477-1483.

[37] Fatima a, Ferreira Juliana C. et al. Maternal Serum Visfatin at 11-13 Weeks of Gestation in Gestational Diabetes Mellitus. Clinical Chemistry 2011 57 609-613.

[38] Kuzmicki M, Telejko B, Szamatowicz J et al. High resistin and interleukin-6 levels are associated with gestational diabetes mellitus. Gynecological Endocrinology 2009 25 258-263.

[39] Cortelazzi D, Corbetta S, Ronzoni S, Pelle F, Marconi A, Cozzi V, Cetin I, Cortelazzi R, Beck-Peccoz P, Spada A. Maternal and foetal resistin and adiponectin concentrations in normal and complicated pregnancies. Clin Endocrinol (Oxf). 2007;66(3):447-453.

[40] Megia A, Vendrell J, Gutierrez C, Sabaté M, Broch M, Fernández-Real J-M, et al. Insulin sensitivity and resistin levels in gestational diabetes mellitus and after parturition. Eur J Endocrinol. 2008; 158:173-178.

[41] Lain KY, Daftary A R, Ness R B et al. First trimester adipocytokine concentrations and risk of developing gestational diabetes later in pregnancy. Clinical Endocrinology 2008 69 407-411.

[42] Yang RZ, Lee MJ, Hu H, Pray J, Wu HB, Hansen BC, Shuldiner AR, Fried SK, McLenithan JC, Gong DW. Identification of omentin as a novel depot-specific adipokine in human adipose tissue: possible role in modulating insulin action. Am J Physiol Endocrinol Metab. 2006;290(6):E12.

[43] Abell SK, Shorakae S, Harrison CL, Hiam D, Moreno-Asso A, Stepto NK, et al. The association between dysregulated adipocytokines in early pregnancy and development of gestational diabetes. Diabetes Metab Res Rev. 2017;33(8):e2926.

[44] Supák D, Melczer Z, Cseh K. Elevated serum acylated (biologically active) ghrelin and resistin levels associate with pregnancy-induced weight gain, insulin resistance and antropometric data in the fetus. Eur J Obstet Gynecol Reprod Biol 2016;206:e111.

[45] Cawthorn WP, Sethi JK. TNF-alpha and adipocyte biology. FEBS Letters 2008 582 117-131.

[46] Gao XL, Yang HX, Zhao Y. Variations of tumor necrosis factor-alpha, leptin and adiponectin in mid-trimester of gestational diabetes mellitus. Chinese Medical Journal 2008 121 701-705.

[47] Xu J, Zhao Y H, Chen Y P et al. Maternal Circulating Concentrations of Tumor Necrosis Factor-Alpha, Leptin, and Adiponectin in Gestational Diabetes Mellitus: A Systematic Review and Meta-Analysis. Scientific World Journal 2014 2014 926-932.

[48] Briana D D, Malamitsi-Puchner A et al Adipocytokines in Normal and

Complicated Pregnancies. Reproductive Sciences 2009 16 921-937.)

[49] Georgiou H M, Lappa M, Georgiou GM, Marita A et al. Screening for biomarkers predictive of gestational diabetes mellitus. Acta Diabetologica 2008 45 157-165.

[50] Kirwan J P, Mouzon S H, Lepercq J et al. TNF-α Is a Predictor of Insulin Resistance in Human Pregnancy. Diabetes 2002 51 2207-2213.

[51] Morisset AS, Dubé MC, Côté JA et al. Circulating interleukin-6 concentrations during and after gestational diabetes mellitus. Acta Obstetricia et Gynecologica Scandinavica 2011 90 524-530.

[52] Wolf M, Sauk J, Shah A et al. Inflammation and glucose intolerance: a prospective study of gestational diabetes mellitus. Diabetes Care 2004 27 21-27.

[53] Georgiou H, Lappas M, Georgiou G M et al. Screening for Biomarkers Predictive of Gestational Diabetes Mellitus. Acta Diabetologica 2008 45 157-165

[54] Prenatal Diagnosis 2011 31 135-141.). Adding maternal visfatin and adiponectin to a set of maternal risk factors resulted in a detection rate of 68% (95% CI: 58.3-76.3%).

[55] O'Malley E G, Ciara Reynoldsa C M E, Killaleab A et al. /European Journal of Obstetrics & Gynecology and Reproductive Biology 250 (2020) 101-106.

[56] Beis C, Grigorakis SI, Philippou G, Alevizaki M, Anastasiou E. Lack of suppression of plasma glucagon levels in late pregnancy persists postpartum only in women with previous gestational diabetes mellitus. Acta Diabetol 2005;42(1):31-35.

[57] Akinci B, Demir T, Saygili S, Yener, Alaccioglu I, Saygili F, et al. Gestational diabetes has no additional effect on plasma thrombin-activatable fibrinolysis inhibitor antigen levels beyond pregnancy. Diabetes Res Clin Pract 2008;81 (1):93-96.

[58] Li G, Kong L, Zhang L, Fan L, Su Y, Rose J, et al. Early pregnancy maternal lipid profiles and the risk of gestational diabetes mellitus stratified for body mass index. Reprod Sci. 2014;22: 712-717.

[59] Correa P J, Venegas P, Palmeiro Y, Albers D, Rice G, Roa J et al. First trimester prediction of gestational diabetes mellitus using plasma biomarkers: a case-control study. J. Perinat. Med. 2018; aop,1-8.

[60] Lorenzo-Almorós A, Hang T, Peiró C et al. Predictive and diagnostic biomarkers for gestational diabetes and its associated metabolic and cardiovascular diseases Cardiovasc Diabetol (2019) 18:140.

[61] Ding EL, Song Y, Malik VS, Liu S. Sex Differences of endogenous sex hormones and risk of type 2 diabetes: a systematic review and metaanalysis. JAMA. 2006;295(11):12.

[62] Smirnakis KV, Plati A, Wolf M, Thadhani R, Ecker JL. Predicting gestational diabetes: choosing the optimal early serum marker. Am J Obstet Gynecol. 2007;196:410.e1-6 (discussion 410.e6-7).

[63] Zhang T, Du T, Li W, Yang S, Liang W. Sex hormone-binding globulin levels during the first trimester may predict gestational diabetes mellitus development. Biomark Med. 2018;12(3):239.

[64] Nanda S, Savvidou M, Syngelaki A, Akolekar R, Nicolaides KH. Prediction of gestational diabetes mellitus by maternal factors and biomarkers at 11 to 13 weeks. Prenat Diagn. 2011;31(2): 135-141.

[65] Kralisch S, Hoffmann A, Lössner U, Kratzsch J, Blüher M, Stumvoll M, et al. Regulation of the novel adipokines/ hepatokines fetuin A and fetuin B in gestational diabetes mellitus. Metab Clin Exp. 2017; 68:88-94.

[66] Kansu-Celik H, Ozgu-Erdinc AS, Kisa B, Findik RB, Yilmaz C, Tasci Y. Prediction of gestational diabetes mellitus in the first trimester: comparison of maternal fetuin-A, N-terminal proatrial natriuretic peptide, high-sensitivity C-reactive protein, and fasting glucose levels. Arch Endocrinol Metab. 2019; 63:121-127.

[67] Bonakdaran S, Khorasani ZM, Jafarzadeh F. Increased serum level of FGF21 in gestational diabetes mellitus. Acta Endocrinol (Buchar).2017; 13:278-81.

[68] Köninger A, Mathan A, Mach P, Frank M, Schmidt B, Schleussner E, et al. Is afamin a novel biomarker for gestational diabetes mellitus? A pilot study. Reprod Biol Endocrinol. 2018;16:30.

[69] Näf S, Escote X, Ballesteros M, Yañez RE, Simón-Muela I, Gil P, Albaiges G, Vendrell J, Megia A. Serum activin A and follistatin levels in gestational diabetes and the association of the activin a-follistatin system with anthropometric parameters in offspring. PLoS ONE. 2014;9(4): e92175.

[70] Poirier C, Desgagné V, Guérin R, Bouchard L. MicroRNAs in pregnancy and gestational diabetes mellitus: emerging role in maternal metabolic regulation. Curr Diabetes Rep. 2017; 17:35.

[71] Morales-Prieto DM, Ospina-Prieto S, Schmidt A, Chaiwangyen W, Markert UR. Elsevier trophoblast research award lecture: origin, evolution and future of placenta miRNAs. Placenta. 2014;35(Suppl): S39–S45.

[72] Zhao C, Dong J, Jiang T, Shi Z, Yu B, Zhu Y, Chen D, Xu J, Huo R, Dai J, Xia Y, Pan S, Hu ZSJ. Early second-trimester serum miRNA profiling predicts gestational diabetes mellitus. PLoS ONE. 2011;6(8): e2392.

[73] Wander PL, Boyko EJ, Hevner K, Parikh VJ, Tadesse MG, Sorensen Teat al. Circulating early- and mid-pregnancy microRNAs and risk of gestational diabetes. Diabetes Res Clin Pract. 2017; 132:1-9.

[74] Hu J, Zhang A, Yang S et al. Combined effects of sex hormone-binding globulin and sex hormones on risk of incident type 2 diabetes. Journal of Diabetes 2015 8 508-515.

[75] Bartha JL, Comino-Delgado R, Romero-Carmona R et al. Sex hormone-binding globulin in gestational diabetes. Acta Obstetricia et Gynecologica Scandinavica 2000 79 839-845.

[76] Maged AM, Moety GAF, Mostafa W A et al. Comparative study between different biomarkers for early prediction of gestational diabetes mellitus. Journal of Maternal-Fetal & Neonatal Medicine 2014 27 1108-1112.

[77] Caglar GS, Ozdemir ED, Cengiz SD et al. Sex-hormone-binding globulin early in pregnancy for the prediction of severe gestational diabetes mellitus and related complications. Journal of Obstetrics and Gynaecology Research 2012 38 1286-1293.

[78] Smirnakis K V, Plati A, Wolf M et al. ,Predicting gestational diabetes: choosing the optimal early serum marker. American Journal of Obstetrics and Gynecology 2007 196 410.e1-410.

[79] Kralisch S, Fasshauer M. Adipocyte fatty acid binding protein: a novel adipokine involved in the pathogenesis of metabolic and vascular disease? Diabetologia 2013 56 10-21.

[80] Ortega-Senovilla H, Schaefer-Graf U, Meitzner K et al. Serum levels of adipocyte fatty acid binding protein are increased in gestational diabetes mellitus. Diabetes Care 2011 34 2061-2066.

[81] Kralisch S, Stepan H, Kratzsch J, Verlohren M et al. Serum levels of adipocyte fatty acid binding protein are increased in gestational diabetes mellitus. European Journal of Endocrinology 2009 160 33-38.

[82] Wu LE, Samocha-Bonet D, Whitworth PT, Fazakerley DJ, Turner N, Biden TJ, et al. Identification of fatty acid binding protein 4 as an adipokine that regulates insulin secretion during obesity. Mol Metab. 2014;3:465-473.

[83] Zabetian-Targhi F, Mahmoudi MJ, Rezaei N, Mahmoudi M. Retinol binding protein 4 in relation to diet, inflammation, immunity, and cardiovascular diseases. Adv Nutr. 2015;6:748-762.

[84] Li YY, Xiao R, Li CP, Huangfu J, Mao JF. Increased plasma levels of FABP4 and PTEN is associated with more severe insulin resistance in women with gestational diabetes mellitus. Med Sci Monit. 2015;8(21):426-431.

[85] Ning H, Tao H, Weng Z, Zhao X. Plasma fatty acid-binding protein 4 (FABP4) as a novel biomarker to predict gestational diabetes mellitus. Acta Diabetol. 2016; 53:891-898.

[86] Du C, Kong F. A prospective study of maternal plasma concentrations of retinol-binding protein 4 and risk of gestational diabetes mellitus. Ann Nutr Metab. 2019; 74:1-8.

[87] Dias S, Pheiffer C, Abrahams Y et al. Int. J. Mol. Sci. 2018, 19, 2926; doi:10.3390/ijms19102926,

[88] Snyder B M, Baer R J, Oltman S C et al. Early pregnancy prediction of gestational diabetes mellitus risk using prenatal screening biomarkers in nulliparous women. Diabetes Research and Clinical Practice 163(2020)108139

[89] Lacroix M, Battista MC, Doyon M. et al. Lower vitamin D levels at first trimester are associated with higher risk of developing gestational diabetes mellitus. Acta Diabetologica 2014 51 609-616.

[90] Zhang M, Pan G, Guo. et al Vitamin D Deficiency Increases the Risk of Gestational Diabetes Mellitus: A Meta-Analysis of Observational Studies. Nutrients 2015 7 8366-8375.

[91] Zhao D, Liming Shen L, Wei Y, Xie J, Chen S, Liang Y et al. Identification of candidate biomarkers for the prediction of gestational diabetes mellitus in the early stages of pregnancy using iTRAQ quantitative proteomics. Proteomics Clin. Appl. 11, 7-8, 2017, 1600152.

[92] Ding M, Chavarro J, Olsen S et al. Genetic variants of gestational diabetes mellitus: a study of 112 SNPs among 8722 women in two independent populations. Diabetologia. 2018 Aug;61(8):1758-1768.

[93] López-Hernández Y, Herrera-Van Oostdam AS, Toro-Ortiz JC, López JA, Salgado-Bustamante M, Murgu M, et al. Urinary metabolites altered during the third trimester in pregnancies complicated by gestational diabetes mellitus: relationship with potential upcoming metabolic disorders. Int J Mol Sci. 2019; 20:1186.

[94] Leitner M, Fragner L, Danner S, Holeschofsky N, Leitner K, Tischler S, Doerfler H, Bachmann G, Sun X, Jaeger W, Kautzky-Willer A. Combined metabolomic analysis of plasma and urine reveals AHBA, tryptophan and serotonin metabolism as potential risk factors in gestational diabetes mellitus (GDM). Front Mol Biosci. 2017; 21(4):84.

[95] Thériault S, Forest J, Massé J et al. Validation of early risk-prediction models for gestational diabetes based on clinical characteristics. Diabetes Research and Clinical Practice, Volume 103, Issue 3, March 2014, Pages 419-425.

[96] Savvidou M, Nelson S M, Makgoba M et al. First-Trimester Prediction of Gestational Diabetes Mellitus: Examining the Potential of Combining Maternal Characteristics and Laboratory Measures. Diabetes 2010 59 3017-3022.

[97] Wannamethee S G, Sattar N, Rumley A et al. Tissue Plasminogen Activator, von Willebrand Factor, and Risk of Type 2 Diabetes in Older Men Diabetes Care 2008 31 995-1000.

[98] Ferreira F, Rezende J C, Vaikousi E et al. Maternal Serum Visfatin at 11-13 Weeks of Gestation in Gestational Diabetes Mellitus. Clinical Chemistry 2011 57 609-613.

[99] Bentley-Lewis R, Huynh J, Xiong G et al. Metabolomic profiling in the prediction of gestational diabetes mellitus. Diabetologia (2015) 58:1329-1332.

[100] Zhanga Z, Gu C, Fang P et al. Endogenous galanin as a novel biomarker to predict gestational diabetes mellitus. Peptides 54 (2014) 186-189.

[101] Siobhan M, Achamallaha M, O'Loughlin J et al. et al. First trimester serum biomarkers to predict gestational diabetes in a high-risk cohort: Striving for clinically useful thresholds. European Journal of Obstetrics & Gynecology and Reproductive Biology 222 (2018) 7-12.

[102] Maged AM, Moety GA, Mostafa WA et al. Comparative study between different biomarkers for early prediction of gestational diabetes mellitus. J Matern Fetal Neonatal Med, 2014; 27(11): 1108-1112.

[103] Georgiou HM, Lappas M, Georgiou GM et al. Screening for biomarkers predictive of gestational diabetes mellitus. Harry M. Georgiou et al. Acta Diabetol (2008) 45:157-165.

[104] Syngelaki A, Kotecha R, Pastides A et al. First-trimester biochemical markers of placentation in screening for gestational diabetes mellitus. Metabolism. 2015;64(11):1485-1489.

[105] Ong CY, Lao TT, Spencer KJ et al. Maternal serum level of placental growth factor in diabetic pregnancies. Reprod Med. 2004;49(6):477-480,

[106] Eleftheriades M, Papastefanou I, Lambrinoudaki I et al. Elevated placental growth factor concentrations at 11-14 weeks of gestation to predict gestational diabetes mellitus. Metabolism. 2014;63(11):1419-1425.

[107] Yarrington CD, Cantonwine DE, Seely EW et al. The Association of Alanine Aminotransferase in Early Pregnancy with Gestational Diabetes. Metab Syndr Relat Disord.2016; 14(5):254-258.

[108] Rasanen J1, Snyder CK, Rao PV et al. Glycosylated fibronectin as a first-trimester biomarker for prediction of gestational diabetes. Obstet Gynecol. 2013;122(3):586-94.

[109] Watanabe N, Morimoto S, Fujiwara T et al Prediction of gestational diabetes mellitus by soluble (pro)renin receptor during the first trimester. J Clin Endocrinol Metab. 2013;98(6):2528-2535.

[110] Syngelaki A, Visser GH, Krithinakis K et al. First trimester screening for gestational diabetes mellitus by maternal factors and markers of inflammation. Metabolism. 2016;65(3):131-137.

[111] Donovan BM, Nidey NL, Jasper EA, Robinson JG, Bao W, Saftlas AF, et al. (2018) First trimester prenatal screening biomarkers and gestational diabetes mellitus: A systematic review and meta-analysis. PLoS ONE 13(7): e0201319. https://doi.org/10.1371/journal.pone.0201319.

[112] Tenenbaum-Gavish K, Sharabi-Nov A, Binyamin D, Møller H J, Danon D, Rothman L et al. First trimester biomarkers for prediction of gestational diabetes mellitus. Placenta 101 (2020) 80-89.

Chapter 2

Epigenetic: New Insight in Gestational Diabetes Mellitus

Maria Grazia Dalfrà, Silvia Burlina and Annunziara Lapolla

Abstract

Gestational diabetes mellitus (GDM) is the more frequent metabolic complication of pregnancy with a prevalence that is significantly increased in the last decade accounting for 12–18% of all pregnancies. Recent evidences strongly suggests that epigenetic profile changes could be involved in the onset of GDM and its related maternal and fetal complications. In particular, the unfavorable intrauterine environment related to hyperglycemia, a feature of GDM, has been evidenced to exert a negative impact on the establishment of the epigenome of the offspring. Furthermore the adverse in utero environment could be one of the mechanisms engaged in the development of adult chronic diseases. The purpose of this article is to review a number of published studies to fill the gap in our understanding of how maternal lifestyle and intrauterine environment influence molecular modifications in the offspring, with an emphasis on epigenetic alterations.

Keywords: gestational diabetes, epigenetic, maternal complications, fetal complications

1. Introduction

Gestational diabetes mellitus (GDM), defined as a glucose intolerance developing or first recognized during pregnancy that is not clearly overt diabetes [1], is increasingly worldwide due mainly to a rising rates of obesity [2–7].

GDM, if not properly diagnosed and/or treated can lead to adverse outcomes for the mother and the child both during and after pregnancy [8–10]. Of note women experiencing GDM and their children are at high risk to develop cardiometabolic diseases (type 2 diabetes, obesity, hyperlipemia, metabolic syndrome, hypertension, cardiovascular disease) later in life [8–10].

Insulin resistance and beta-cell disfunction are the main physiopathological mechanisms involved in GDM development [4–7]. However all the actors involved are not completely understood as an intricate network of metabolic pathways work in pregnancy complicated by GDM, that includes an abnormal expression of proteins involved in glucose and lipid metabolism, inflammation, oxidative stress, immune response, organ development, and cell death regulation. In this context recent studies have suggested that genetic, epigenetic and environmental factors contributes in GDM development [11–14], (**Figure 1**). In addition, the adverse intrauterine environment in patients with GDM could also have a negative impact on the establishment of the epigenomes of the offspring [15, 16].

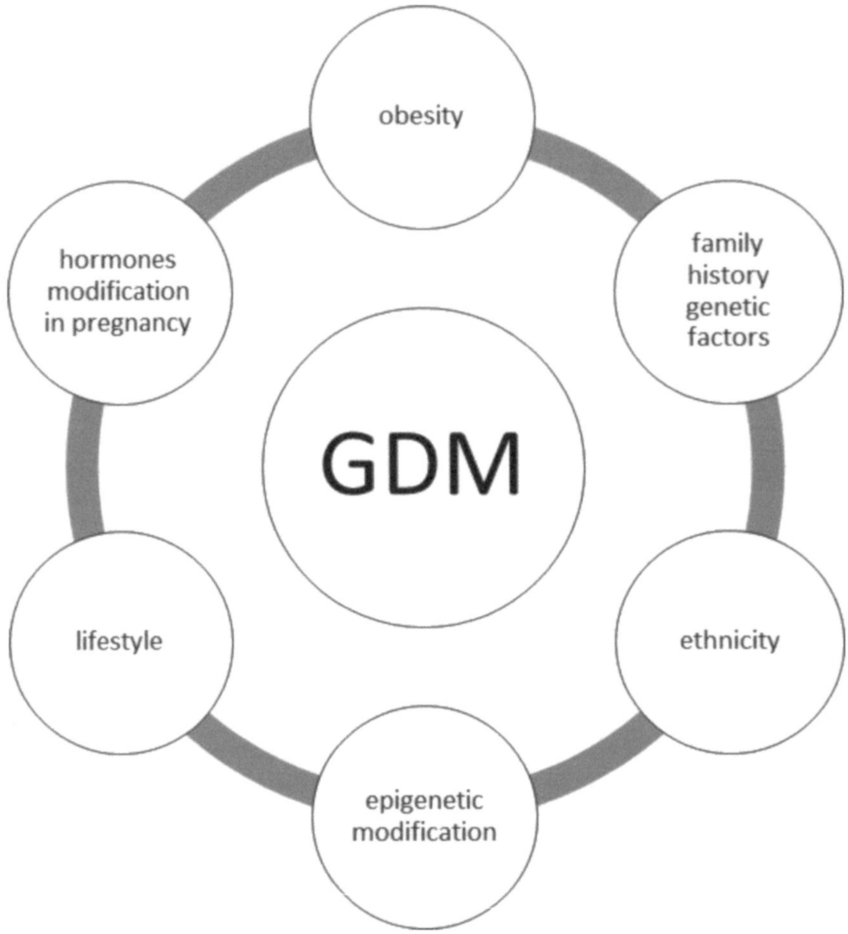

Figure 1.
Factors contributing to GDM development.

The purpose of this article is to review a number of published studies to fill the gap in our understanding how the intrauterine environment can determine molecular modifications in the offspring, with an emphasis on epigenetic alterations.

2. Epigenetic: the meaning

Epigenetic is the study of changes in gene expression caused by mechanisms not involving variations in DNA sequences but determining changes as DNA methylation, histone modifications, and messenger RNA (mRNA) binding by microRNAs (miRNAs).

The study of epigenetic modifications can therefore be useful in deepening and clarifying the pathogenesis of GDM as well as in the use of markers for diagnosis, risk prediction and follow up of different types of pathologies as GDM.

Methylation of cytosine on CpG in the DNA so determining the formation of methylcytosine (5-mc) is the first studied DNA modification. Methylation can determine an increased gene expression by silencing some repressor elements, but, in some regions of DNA as the promoter ones, it can reduce gene expression by inhibiting the activity of enhancer elements [17].

Histone modification can influence the gene expression by modifying the chromatin packing [18].

Micro RNAas are small non-coding single stranded RNAs of about 22 nucleotides that are involved in post-trancriptional regulation of gene expression. It has been evidenced that miRNAs can affect the stability and translation of RNA [19]. Interestingly, some recently-identified miRNAs have been associated with insulin secretion, insulin resistance, and inflammation in patients affected by type 2 diabetes [14].

3. Epigenetic and GDM

It has been demonstrated that even slight increases in glycemia can be associated with epigenetic adaptations via the so-called "metabolic memory", and in this context few studies have examined the association between methylation and GDM development. Of note Whu and coworkers firstly identified two differently methylated genes in plasma, umbilical cord and placenta samples of pregnant women that develop GDM, the Hook Microtubule Tethering Protein 2 (HOOK2), and Retinol Dehydrogenase 12 (RDH12). HOOK2 is a protein that mediates binding to organelles, and is involved in cilia morphogenesis and endocytosis. RDH12 encodes a retinal reductase involved in short-chain aldehyde metabolism [20] (**Tables 1** and **2**).

In this frame more studies have been performed evaluating microRNA: Zhao and coworkers [21], evidenced that the expression of miR222, miR-132 and miR-29a was significantly lower in women who were diagnosed as affected by GDM at 24–28 WG with respect to non GDM control pregnant women. MiR-29 has a role in glucose homeostasis, in particular when overexpressed reduce the insulin-stimulated glucose uptake and the gluconeogenesis [22]. MiR-132 is involved in the regulation of cytochrome P450,mediated by insulin, furthermore when its expression is reduced impairs the correct development of trophoblast, [14, 22].

Successively, as omental adipose tissue is known to play a role in insulin resistance in GDM, the differential expression patterns of miRNAs in omental adipose tissues from GDM patients and pregnant women with normal glucose tolerance was studied [23]. MiR-222 was found to be significantly up-regulated in GDM by quantitative real-time PCR and its expression was related with serum estradiol levels, whereas the expressions of estrogen receptor (ER)-α protein and insulin-sensitive membrane transporter glucose transporter 4 (GLUT4) protein were markedly reduced. Then in order to silence miR-222 in 3 T3-L1 adipocytes the antisense transfection oligonucleotides of miR-222 was applied. An important increase of the expressions of ERα and GLUT4, the insulin-stimulated translocation of GLUT4 from the cytoplasm to the cell membrane and of the uptake of glucose was evidenced in mature adipocites. On the basis of their results the authors conclude that: "miR-222 is a potential regulator of ERα expression in estrogen-induced insulin resistance in GDM and could be a candidate biomarker and therapeutic target for GDM".

Cao and coworkers [24], in 85 pregnant women with GDM found that the relative and absolute expression of plasma microRNA-16-5p, −17-5p, −20a-5p were significantly upregulated, with respect to 72 pregnant women without GDM. During pregnancy, the expression of those microRNAs from GDM women were also positively correlated with insulin resistance. Furthermore, significative differences were found in GDM women with respect to normal pregnant ones in the plasma levels of microRNA-16-5p, −17-5p, −20a-5p and in the areas under the curve (0.92, 0.88, and 0.74, respectively). The authors conclude that plasma microRNA-16-5p, −17-5p and -20a-5p are potential diagnostic biomarkers in GDM. MiR16.5

	Gene	Authors
Mothers	**HOOK2**	WHU, 2016
	RDH12	Whu,2016
	H3K27	Michialczy 2016
	H3K4	Michialczy 2016
Placenta	**ADIPOQ**	Bouchard 2010
	TNFRSF1B	Cardenas 2018
	LDLR	Cardenas2018
	BLM	Cardenas 2018
	PDE4B	Cardenas 2018
	ABCA1	Houde 2013
	MEST	Hajj 2018
	NR3C1	Hajj 2018
Offspring	**NR3C1**	Hajj 2018
	PYGO1	Allard 2015
	CLN8	Allard 2015
	PRDM16	Côté 2016
	BMP7	Côté 2016
	PPARGC1a	Côté 2016
	MEST	Hajj 2018
	ATPSA1	Haerle 2017
	NFAP4	Haerle 2017
	PRKCH	Haerle 2017
	SLC17A	Haerle 2017

Table 1.
Gene methylation in gestational diabetes mellitus.

is implicated in the insulin sensitivity regulation and it is upregulated in type 2 diabetes. MiR17–5 has a role is the proliferation of smooth muscle cell. MiR20a-5p is upregulated in preeclampsia, a well known complication of diabetic pregnancy.

Wander and coworkers [25] analyzed the role of miRNA in women affected by GDM and different body mass index. MiR155-5p, and 21–3p were found positively associated with GDM. The miR-21-3p and miR-210-3p were positively associate only in GDM overweight/obese women. MiR-155 and MiR21–3 have a role in pathways that regulate cell survival, and inflammation. MiR210-3p is associated with angiogenesis [14].

As for histone modification, Michalczyk and coworkers [26], analyzed several epigenetic markers during and after pregnancy in a small, multiethnic population. The evaluation of the proportion of total H3 histone methylated GDM women who developed type 2 diabetes after pregnancy showed a significantly lower H3K27 (50%)with respect to non-diabetic women; furthermore type2 diabetic women with previous GDM had also significantly lower H3K4 (75%) with respect to GDM with normal glucose tolerance after pregnancy. A study evaluating a large sample size for a longer post partum follow up is however necessary to confirm that histone methylation could be a useful predictor of type 2 diabetes in women with GDM.

	miRNA	miRNA impaired	Author
Mothers	**miR-132**	Reduced expression	Zhou et al. 2019 Zhao et al. 2011
	miR29a	Reduced expression	Zhao et al. 2011
	miR222	Reduced expression	Zhao et al. 2011
	miR16-5p	Up-regulation	Cao et al. 2017
	miR17–5p	Up-regulation	Cao et al. 2017
	miR20a-5p	Up-regulation	Cao et al. 2017
	miR 155-5p	Overexpression	Wander et al. 2017
	miR 21–3p	Overexpression	Wander et al. 2017
	miR210-3p	Overexpressiion	Wander et al. 2017
Placenta	**miR98**	Up-regulation	Cao et al. 2016

Table 2.
Studies assessing the role of mRNAs in gestational diabetes.

4. Epigenetic and placenta

The placenta undergoes a number of structural and functional changes in pregnant women affected by diabetes due to the increased production of inflammatory cytokines determined by the high levels of maternal glucose [27]. In this frame, utilizing different mass spectrometry approaches - such as MALDI-MS and LC-MS^E – in the evaluation of placental samples from women with and without GDM, it has been showed that if well controlled, GDM induces only minor changes in the placental proteome [28]. So it is of interest to verify if epigenetic modifications can however occur at the placental level even with relatively low maternal glucose levels and if the extent of these modifications is in some way related to glycemic levels (**Tables 1** and **2**).

Lesseur and coworkers investigate the relations between prepregnancy obesity and GDM and placental leptin DNA methylation on 535 mother-neonate enrolled in the Rhode Island Child health Study. The results of the study showed that neonates of mothers affected by GDM had higher placenta leptin methylation levels similar to those of the mothers with prepregnancy obesity. So maternal metabolic milieu before and during pregnancy can determine impairment of placenta methylation so contributing to the metabolic fetal programming of obesity [29]. These data well fit with those reported by Bouchard et al. [30]. In a subsequent paper Bouchard et al. [31], evaluated the possible association between the methylation of adiponectin gene (ADIPOQ) in plasma cord blood and placenta tissue and plasma glucose levels of pregnant women. They found low DNA methylation levels in the ADIPOQ promoter on the fetal side of the placenta that were positively related with high maternal glucose levels in the second trimester of pregnancy. Furthermore, the low DNA methylation levels on the maternal side of the placenta were also positively related to insulin resistance, assessed with the homeostasis model assessment method (HOMA), and to high circulating adiponectin levels during pregnancy.

Furthermore, a negative correlation between DNA methylation of the ATP-binding cassette transporter A1 (ABCA1) gene on the placenta maternal site and HDL and 2 hour OGTT plasma glucose was found in 26 GDM women. When looking at the placenta fetal site, DNA methylation of ABCA1 was negatively associated with cord blood tryglicerides [32].

In a well conducted study, Cao et al. aim to verify the role of miRNA-98 in placental tissues from GDM patients, considering that MiRNA-98 is implicated in the correct embryo implantation [33]. They showed that, in the placentas of GDM patients miR-98 is upregulated and total DNA methylation levels are reduced with respect to normal pregnant women. These results,considering that MiRNA-98 regulates the Mecp2 target gene a key protein for embrio development, coud have important consequences for fetal growth.

More recently Cardenas and coworkers [34] conducted an elegant epigenome-wide association study (involving 850,000 CpG sites) on samples of placenta and plasma glucose, and related them to 2 h post-OGTT plasma glucose levels in 448 mother-and-infant pairs at 24–30 weeks of gestation. They found a lower DNA methylation of 4 CpG sites within the phosphodiesterase 4b gene that are positively correlated with plasma glucose at 2 h OGTT. Furthermore, a differentially methylation behavior in relation with maternal glucose was found for 3 CpG sites in the TNFRSF1B, LDLR and BLM.

DNA methylation correlated with expression of its respective genes in placental tissue at three out of four independent identified loci:PDE4B, TNFRSF1B, and LDLR. TNFRSF1B is involved in apoptosis, LDLR encodes a lipoprotein receptor that mediates LDL endocytosis in the cells, and is also expressed in the placenta. BLM is associated with genome stability and maintenance. So maternal glycemic levels during pregnancy were associated with placental DNA methylation of inflammatory genes, the expression of which depends on epigenetic changes.

5. Epigenetic and offspring

The Developmental Origins of Health and Disease, largely derived from the Barker hypothesis [16], strongly suggests that not only undernutrition but also overnutrition, maternal obesity and diabetes can determine chronic diseases in the offspring through an early exposure to a suboptimal fetal environment; in this context epigenetic modifications have been showed to contribute mainly to this (**Table 1**).

Hajj et al. [35], have evaluated the effect of GDM on the epigenome of the offspring. To reach this aim they analyzed cord blood and placental tissue from the newborn of GDM patients 88 of them treated with diet and 98 with insulin. The results of the study show meaningful lower methylation levels in GDM compared with pregnant women without GDM in the levels of the maternal imprinting MEST gene and the non-imprinting glucocorticoid receptor NR3C1 gene. It is to notice that these genes are associated with placental and fetal growth. Low levels of MEST methylation have also been found in plasma of adults with obesity with respect to normal-weight controls. So the intrauterine exposure to GDM has effects on the epigenome of the offspring, and epigenetic malprogramming of MEST can contribute to predisposing individuals to obesity later in life.

The effect of the exposure to maternal diabetes in utero has been investigated by a genome-wide methylation analysis on peripheral mononuclear cell's DNA in 21 healthy children of GDM mothers, by utilizing a mediation analysis [36]. A series of genes have been identified to be associated with cardiometabolic risk among that the ubiquitin proteasome system (UPS) was the most important. An increased methylation of PYGO1 and CLN 8 showed the most important mediation effect on VCAM-1 levels of the children. TheVCAM-1 protein mediates the adhesion of lymphocytes, monocytes, eosinophils, and basophils to vascular endothelium. It also functions in leukocyte-endothelial cell signal transduction, and it may play a role in the development of atherosclerosis.

A 2 step epigenetic Mendelian randomization approach was used by Allard et al. on data of 485 mothers and their children [37]. To take into consideration maternal glycemia, a genetic risk score, based on 10 known genetic variant related to glycemia, was firstly developed (GRs 10). The results of the study showed that an high GRs 10 was associated with a lower methylation of cg 12083122 that is located near the leptin gene. The low methylation levels at cg12083122 was associated with high cord leptin levels, so evidencing that maternal glycemia can influence offspring leptin epigenetic modulation. In this frame, to evaluate the possible relation of maternal hyperglycemia and DNA methylation of genes involved in brown adipose tissue activation, the DNA methylation levels were measured in placenta samples from normal and GDM women and compared to results of maternal plasma glucose levels. The values of maternal plasma glucose, at the second and third trimester of pregnancy, resulted correlated with the methylation levels of PRDM16, BMP 7 and PPARGC1a and with cord blood leptin levels. These results suggest that maternal glycemia can determine modification in genes related to obesity development in the offsring [38]. More recently, an Illumina 450 K methylation arrays was utilized to analyze genome-wide methylation patterns in fetal cord blood of pregnant women with and without GDM. Significant differences in methylation were found between the GDM patients and the normal pregnant women; furthermore, these differences were more significant in GDM women treated with insulin. A series of genes were found modified by methylation and in particular: ATPSA1, which encodes a subunit of mitochondrial ATP synthetase that acts also reducing mitochondrial oxidation; MFAP4, which is engaged in the process of cell adhesion and intercellular interaction; PRKCH, a component of the protein C family engaged in numerous signaling pathways; and SLC17A, or sodium/phosphate cotransporter involved in hypoxia events. It is to emphasize that these methylation modifications even if had a small effect size, affects many genes/loci [39]. Furthermore, methylation that affects a series of genes that can impair insulin secretion and increase the risk of diabetes and obesity has been reported in offspring of mother affected by type 2 diabetes a condition that shares the same physiopathological mechanisms of GDM [40].

6. Conclusions

The studies taken into consideration made a significant contribution to the knowledge of the physiopathological basis of GDM and of its complications, however methodological problems, small sample size, different GDM diagnostic criteria, make difficult to have final conclusion.

Further researches with high study power need to be undertaken in order to be more confident on the role of epigenetic in GDM disease, bearing also in mind that epigenetic expression in pregnancy varies with weeks of gestation, sex of the fetus, ethnicity, type of sample considered. These studies must be able to determine new road for intervention so to reduce in GDM patients and their children the development of the chronic metabolic diseases [41, 42].

Abbreviations

GDM	Gestational diabetes mellitus
miRNAs	microRNAs
CpG	C-phosphate-G sites
5-mc	methylcytosine
HOOK2	Hook Microtubule Tethering Protein 2

RDH12	Retinol Dehydrogenase 12
ER	estrogen receptor (ER)-α protein
GLUT4	sodium glucose transporter 4
H3K27	tri-methylation of lysine 27 on histone H3 protein.
H3K4	H3K4 histone
MALDI-MS	Matrix-Assisted Laser Desorption/Ionization Mass Spectrometry
LC-MS^E	Liquid Chromatography / Mass Spectrometry
ADIPOQ	Human Adiponectin, C1Q and Collagen Domain
HOMA	Homeostasis Model Assessment Method
ABCA1	ATP-Binding Cassette Transporter A1
Mecp2	Methyl-CpG Binding Protein 2
TNFRSF1B	TNF Receptor Superfamily Member 1B
LDLR	Low Density Lipoprotein Receptor
BLM	BLM RecQ Like Helicase
MEST	Mesodermic Specific Transcript Gene
NR3C1	Nuclear Receptor Subfamily 3 Group C Member 1
UPS	Ubiquitin Proteasome System
PYGO1	Pygopus Family PHD Finger 1
CLN 8	CLN8 Transmembrane ER and ERGIC Protein
VCAM	Human Vascular Cell Adhesion Molecule 1
GRs 10	Genetic Risk Score
PRDM16	PR Domain Containing 16
BMP 7	Bone Morphogenic Protein 7
PPARGC1a	Peroxisome Proliferator Activated Receptor Gamma
ATPSA1	Subunit of Mitocondrial ATP Synthetase
MFAP4	Microfibril Associated Protein 4
PRKCH	Protein Kinase C family
CTBP2	C-Terminal Binding Protein 2

Author details

Maria Grazia Dalfrà, Silvia Burlina and Annunziara Lapolla*
DPT Medicine-Padova University, Padova, Italy

*Address all correspondence to: annunziata.lapolla@unipd.it

References

[1] International Association of Diabetes and Pregnancy Study Groups Consensus Panel. International Association of Diabetes and Pregnancy Study Groups: Recommendations on the diagnosis and classification of hyperglycemia in pregnancy. Diabetes Care. 2010; 33: 676-668.

[2] Koning SH, Hoogenberg K, Lutgers HL, Van den Berg PP, Wolffenbuttel BHR. Gestational diabetes mellitus: current knowledge and unmet needs. J Diabetes. 2016; 8(6): 770-781.

[3] Lapolla A, Metzger BE. The post-HAPO situation with gestational diabetes: the bright and dark sides. Acta Diabetol. 2018; 55(9):885-892.

[4] Ryan EA, Enns L. Role of gestational hormones in the induction of insulin resistance. J Clin Endocrinol Metab. 1988; 67:341-347.

[5] Kampmann U, Knorr S, Fuglsang J, Ovesen P. Determinants of Maternal Insulin Resistance during Pregnancy: An Updated Overview. J Diabetes Res. 2019 Nov 19;2019:5320156. doi: 10.1155/2019/5320156. PMID: 31828161; PMCID: PMC6885766.

[6] Lain K, Catalano PM. Metabolic changes in pregnancy. Clin Obstet Gynaecol.2007; 50:938- 948.

[7] Lapolla A, Dalfrà MG, Mello G, Parretti E, Cioni R, Marzari C et al. Early detection of insulin sensitivity and beta-cell function with simple tests indicates future derangements in late pregnancy. J Clin Endocrinol Metab. 2008; 93:876-880.

[8] Burlina S, Dalfrà MG, Lapolla A. Short- and long-term consequences for offspring exposed to maternal diabetes: a review. J Matern Fetal Neonatal Med. 2019; 32(4):687-694.

[9] Lowe WL, Scholtens DM, Lowe LP, Kuang A, Nodzenky M, Talbot O et al. Association of gestational diabetes with maternal disorders of glucose metabolism and childhood adiposity. JAMA. 2018;11;320(10):1005-1016.

[10] Burlina S, Dalfrà MG, Lapolla A. Clinical and biochemical approach to predicting post-pregnancy metabolic decompensation. Diabetes Res Clin Pract. 2018;145:178-183.

[11] Whu L, Cui L, Tam WH, Ma RC, Wang CC. Genetic variants associated with gestational diabetes mellitus: a meta-analysis and subgroup analysis. Scientific Reports. 2016; 6: 30539.

[12] Pantham P, Aye IL, Powell T. Inflammation in maternal obesity and gestational diabetes mellitus. Placenta. 2015; 36:709-715.

[13] Lapolla A, Dalfrà MG, Sanzari M, Fedele D, Betterle C, Masin M et al. Lymphocyte subsets and cytokines in women with gestational diabetes mellitus and their newborn. Cytochine. 2005; 31:280-287.

[14] Zhu H, Leung SW. Identification of microRNA biomarkers in type 2 diabetes: a meta-analysis of controlled profiling studies. Diabetologia. 2015; 58: 900-911.

[15] Agarwal P, Morriseau TS, Kereliuk SM, Doucette CA, Wicklow BA, Dolinsky VW. Maternal obesity, diabetes during pregnancy and epigenetic mechanisms that influence the developmental origins of cardiometabolic disease in the offspring. Crit Rev Clin Lab Sci. 2018; Mar;55(2):71-101. doi: 10.1080/10408363.2017.1422109. Epub 2018 Jan 8. PMID: 29308692.

[16] Barker DJ. The fetal and infant origins of adult disease. BMJ. 1990; 301:1111-1122.

[17] Hernando-Herraez I, Garcia-Perez R, Sharp AJ, Marques-Bonet T. DNA Methylation: Insights into Human Evolution. PLoS Genet. 2015; Dec 10;11(12):e1005661. doi: 10.1371/journal.pgen.1005661. PMID: 26658498; PMCID: PMC4684328.

[18] Martin C, Zhang Y. The diverse functions of histone lysine methylation. Nat Rev Mol Cell Biol. 2005 Nov;6(11):838-849. doi: 10.1038/nrm1761. PMID: 16261189.

[19] Zhao S, Liu MF. Mechanisms of microRNA-mediated gene regulation. Sci China C Life Sci. 2009 Dec;52(12):1111-1116. doi: 10.1007/s11427-009-0152-y. Epub 2009 Dec 17. PMID: 20016967.

[20] Whu P, Farrel W E, Haworth K E, Emes RD, Kitchen MO, Glossop JR, Fryer AA. Maternal genome-wide DNA methylation profile in gestational diabetes shows distinctive disease-associated changes relative to matched healthy pregnancies. Epigenetics.2016; 13: 122-128.

[21] Zhao C, Dong J, Jiang T, Shi Z, Yu B, Zhu Y et al. Early second trimester serum miRNA profiling predicts gestational diabetes mellitus. PLoS ONE. 2011: 6:23925-23923.

[22] Zhou X, Xiang C, Zheng X. MiR-132 serves as a diagnostic biomarker in gestational diabetes mellitus and its regulatory effect on trophoblast cell viability. Diagnostic Pathology. 2019; 14:119-128.

[23] Shi Z, Zhao C, Guo X, Ding H, Cui Y, Shen R, Liu J. Differential expression of microRNAs in omental adipose tissue from gestational diabetes mellitus subjects reveals miR-222 as a regulator of ERα expression in estrogen-induced insulin resistance. Endocrinology. 2014; May;155(5):1982-90. doi: 10.1210/en.2013-2046. Epub 2014 Mar 6. PMID: 24601884.

[24] Cao YL, Jia YJ, Xing BH, Shi DD, Dong XJ. Plasma microRNA-16-5p, 17-5p and 20a-5p: novel diagnostic biomarkers for gestational diabetes mellitus. Obstet Gynecol Res 2017; 43:974-981.

[25] Wander PL, Boyko EJ, Hevner K, Parikin VJ, Tadesse MG, Sorensen TK et al. Circulating early- and mid-pregnancy microRNAs and risk of gestational diabetes. Diab Res Clin Pract. 2017; 132:1-9.

[26] Michalczyk AA, Dunbar JA, Janus ED, Best JD, Ebeling PR, Ackland MJ et al. Epigenetic markers to predict conversion from gestational diabetes to type 2 diabetes. J Clin Endocrinol Metab. 2016; 101: 2396-2404.

[27] Hauguel-de Mouzon S, Desoye G The placenta in diabetic pregnancy: new methodological approaches. In Gestational Diabetes: a decade after the HAPO study. Lapolla A, Metzger BE eds, Frontier in Diabetes Karger 2020; pp 145-154.

[28] Burlina S, Banfi C, Brioschi M, Visentin S, Dalfrà MG, Traldi P, Lapolla A. Is the placenta proteome impaired in well-controlled gestational diabetes? J Mass Spectrom. 2019; 54:359-365.

[29] Lesseur C, Armstrong DA, Paquette AG, Li Z, Padbury JF, Marsit CJ. Maternal obesity and gestational diabetes are associated with placental leptin DNA methylation. Am J Obstet Gynecol. 2014; Dec;211(6):654.e1-9. doi: 10.1016/j.ajog.2014.06.037. Epub 2014 Jun 19. PMID: 24954653; PMCID: PMC4254188.

[30] Bouchard L, Thibault S, Guay SP, Santure M, Monpetit A, St-Pierre J et al. Leptin gene epigenetic adaptation to impaired glucose metabolism during pregnancy. Diabetes Care. 2010; Nov;33(11):2436-41. doi: 10.2337/dc10-1024. Epub 2010 Aug 19. PMID: 20724651; PMCID: PMC2963508.

[31] Bouchard L, Hivert M, Guay SP, StPierre J, Perron P, Brisson D. Placental adiponectin gene DNA methylation levels are associated with mother's blood glucose concentration. Diabetes. 2012; 61:1272-1280.

[32] Houde AA, Guay SP, Desgagné V, Hivert MF, Baillargeon JP, St-Pierre J et al. Adaptations of placental and cord blood ABCA1 DNA methylation profile to maternal metabolic status. Epigenetics. 2013; Dec;8(12):1289-302. doi: 10.4161/epi.26554. Epub 2013 Oct 10. PMID: 24113149; PMCID: PMC3933490.

[33] Cao JL, Zhang L, Lin J, Tian S, Lv XD, Wang XQ et al. Up-regulation of miR-98 and unravelling regulatory mechanisms in gestational diabetes mellitus. Sci Rep.2016; 6:32268-32274.

[34] Cardenas A, Gagnè-Quellet V, Allard C, Brisson D, Perron P, Bouchard L et al. Placental DNA methylation adaptation to maternal glycemic response in pregnancy. Diabetes. 2018; 67: 1673-1683.

[35] Hajj NE, Pliushch G, Schneider E, Dittrich M, Muller T, Korenov M et al. Metabolic programming of MEST DNA methylation by intrauterine exposure to gestational diabetes mellitus. Diabetes. 2018; 62: 1320-1328.

[36] West NA, Kechris K, Dabelea D. Exposure to Maternal Diabetes in Utero and DNA Methylation Patterns in the Offspring. Immunometabolism. 2013; Mar;1:1-9. doi: 10.2478/immun-2013-0001. PMID: 23741625; PMCID: PMC3670583.

[37] Allard C, Desgagné V, Patenaude J, Lacroix M, Guillemette L, Battista MC, et al. Mendelian randomization supports causality between maternal hyperglycemia and epigenetic regulation of leptin gene in newborns. Epigenetics. 2015;10(4):342-51. doi: 10.1080/15592294.2015.1029700. PMID: 25800063; PMCID: PMC4622547.

[38] Côté S, Gagné-Ouellet V, Guay SP, Allard C, Houde AA, Perron P et al. PPARGC1α gene DNA methylation variations in human placenta mediate the link between maternal hyperglycemia and leptin levels in newborns. Clin Epigenetics. 2016; Jun 22;8:72. doi: 10.1186/s13148-016-0239-9. PMID: 27340502; PMCID: PMC4918074.

[39] Haerle L, Haj N, Dittrich M, Muller T, Nanda I, Lehnen H. Epigenetic signatures of gestational diabetes mellitus on cord blood methylation. Clinical Epigenetics.2017; 9:28-38.

[40] Chen P, Piaggi P, Traurig M, Bogardus C, Knowler WC, Baier LJ, Hanson RL. Differential methylation of genes in individuals exposed to maternal diabetes in utero. Diabetologia. 2017;Apr;60(4):645-655. doi: 10.1007/s00125-016-4203-1. Epub 2017 Jan 26. PMID: 28127622; PMCID: PMC7194355.

[41] Michels K. Epigenetics epidemiology. 2012. Dondrecht New York Springer Verlag.

[42] Ibarra A, Vega-Guedes B, Brito-Casillas Y, Wagner A Diabetes in pregnancy and microRNAs :promises and limitations in their clinical applications. Non-coding RNA; 2018; 4:1-250.

Chapter 3

The Interaction between the Gut Microbiota and Chronic Diseases

Temitope Sanusi-Olubowale

Abstract

The world is experiencing an increase in chronic diseases like diabetes, inflammatory bowel diseases, cancer, cardiovascular diseases, obesity, and diabetes preceding disease like gestational diabetes. Most of these diseases can be prevented and mitigated if individuals pay attention to the causative factors. One of such factors is the type of microorganisms in an individual's gut. Even though there are innate beneficial microorganisms in the human gut, pathogenic microorganisms can invade the gut, changing the inborn population of the gut microbiota. The changes in the gut microbiota population have been linked to several diseases. This chapter, therefore, describes gut microbiota and their interaction with specific diseases. Also discussed in this chapter are the changes to gut microbiota composition that pose a risk to the host. There is substantial evidence that diseases are initiated or worsened with a change in the gut microbiota composition. Therefore, the gut microbiota plays a crucial role in individuals' health and requires human efforts to keep them in the right population. Furthermore, making lifestyle changes, particularly food choices and behaviors such as the misuse of medications and excessive alcohol consumption, should be monitored and controlled to support gut health.

Keywords: Gut microbiota, Bacteria phylum, Gestational diabetes, Chronic diseases, Gut dysbiosis

1. Introduction

Chronic diseases (CD) are unfavorable health statuses lasting for over one year or more [1, 2]. Such diseases require continual medical attention and activities that could mitigate the severity [1, 2]. The diseases are the leading cause of death and incapacity worldwide, with influences on all socio-economic setups. In 2002, the CD was reported as the cause of 60% of death and 43% global distress [1, 3]. In 2020, the cause of death through CD had risen to 73% and universal distress of 60%, as shown in **Figure 1** [3]. The cause of some of these diseases was attributed to different factors such as genes, poor diet, and lifestyle [1, 4]. The common CD includes diabetes, cancer, cardiovascular diseases, chronic pulmonary diseases, obesity, arthritis, stroke, Alzheimer's diseases, chronic kidney diseases, inflammatory bowel diseases, tooth decay, and epilepsy [1, 3, 5]. Some diseases are signals to the potential development of chronic diseases. Women who have gestational diabetes are at risk of developing type 2 diabetes, hypertension, cardiovascular diseases, and obesity, just as high blood cholesterol could be indicative of future coronary heart diseases, obesity, and hypertension [6, 7].

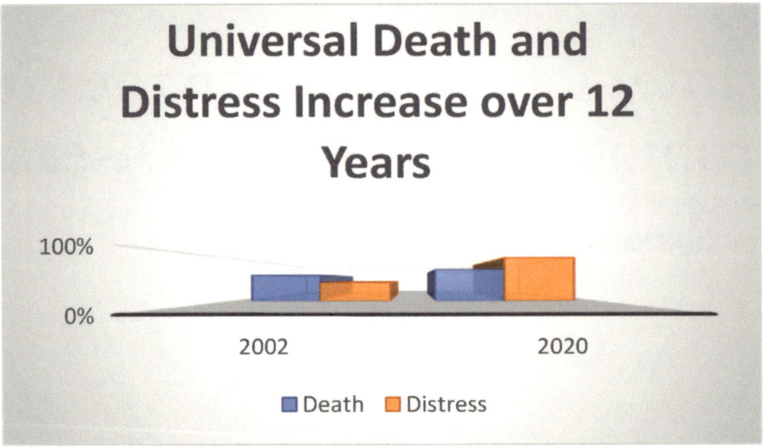

Figure 1.
Chart showing the rate of increase in death and distress as caused by chronic diseases.

Asides from death and health difficulties associated with CD, there are several negative impacts socially and economically. The family of people suffering from one or more CD reported increased personal life burden, financial difficulties, impaired social relations, and intrinsic rewards [8, 9]. Likewise, treating CD and helping people with such diseases significantly impact different countries' finances. It has become a substantial financial burden to nations [10, 11]. In the United States of America, $327 billion is spent annually on medical costs for diabetes [5]. About $147 billion per year for the health cost of obesity, $164 billion for arthritis, $500 billion for Alzheimer's diseases, epilepsy takes $8.6 billion annually, and $45 billion is spent on annual health care for tooth decay [5]. In 2015, a forecasted percentage of Gross Domestic Product (GDP) loss was reported for different countries worldwide. Brazil was expected to lose 3.21% of GDP, Canada, 0.64%, China, 3.94%, India, 5.05%, Nigeria, 3.07%, Russia, 12.35%, Tanzania, 4.19%, United Kingdom, 5.18% GDP losses from death caused by diseases. In another report, the United States loses $1.1trillion annually from the lack of productivity of citizens living with CD. Reducing the rate of obesity alone in the country would increase productivity by $254 billion and $60 billion in reductions in treatment costs [10, 11].

With the national, family, and personal losses associated with CD, methods of curbing the rising rate call for more research, government and non-governmental initiatives, and policies [10]. One research aspect was to figure out the genesis of all these diseases [4, 12]. From different findings, diverse components contribute to the incidence of diseases or increase the risks of developing these diseases. For example, the cause of some of these diseases was attributed to individual genes, other influences such as unhealthy diet, overweight, sedentary lifestyle (lack of physical activities), and risk behaviors such as tobacco use and excessive alcohol were identified. One crucial discovery on factors contributing to disease incidence was the gut microbiota [13–15].

2. The gut microbiota

The human body consists of several microorganisms which were innately beneficial to the host. These colonies of microorganisms that have settled in the human's gastrointestinal tract (GIT, gut) over many years include bacteria, eukaryotes, bacteriophages, archaea, and fungi, and they are called the gut microbiota (GM) [13, 16]. The GM has evolved and established a commensal relationship with the human host over many years. Hence, they are equally referred to as commensals microorganisms because they provide health benefits to the host while the commensals get nutrients from the host without harming the host [13, 16].

There are trillions of microorganisms colonizing humans, but research focuses on the bacteria community [17, 18]. Some years ago, scientists reported that the bacteria cells in the GIT are numerous, much more than the number of cells in the body. Some other researchers claimed that the bacterial cells in the GIT are ten times more than body cells [13, 19]. Recent studies, however, showed human cells and bacterial cells are at a ratio of 1:1 [13, 19, 20].

Humans' GM is developed from birth [19, 21, 22]. Particularly for babies delivered vaginally, the microbiota in the mother's cervix is passed on to the babies. This GM received from birth builds the first wall of defense in children, and the population of GM gradually changes as the child grows. In addition, gut bacteria aid adaptive immunity, a crucial function of the GM in the human's body [13, 21, 22].

2.1 Functions of gut microbiota

The GM proffer benefits to the host. The first known function is to assist in building immunity after birth. The GM has other functions in the body; they contribute advantages anatomically, physiologically, and immunologically [19, 23].

2.1.1 Anatomical and physiological functions

The GM is known for the breakdown of carbohydrates, particularly the indigestible dietary fibers, like cellulose, resistant starch, pectin, oat, wheat bran, and inulin [24, 25]. The absorption of nutrients from dietary fiber has been associated with satiety feeling after eating, thus preventing overeating. The GM metabolizes protein by the secretion of digestive enzymes. Synthesis of vitamin K and B vitamins such as vitamin B12, riboflavin, niacin, and folate, and other digestive enzymes are also performed by GM [23, 24]. The GM also performs physiological benefits of strengthening the gut, shaping the intestinal epithelium, and harvesting energy [13].

Anatomically, the GM assists in maintaining the mucosal barrier's strength by shaping the intestinal epithelium, thereby sustaining gut integrity. Furthermore, the metabolites produced during the breakdown of dietary fibers are absorbed by the epithelial cells to assist cell proliferation, differentiation, and apoptosis of harmful cells, like the cancer cells [23, 26]. The GM is sometimes called the second brain because of its effect on the brain. This is because the metabolites released during the breakdown of fibers are absorbed to support brain activities [19, 27].

2.1.2 Immunological functions

The GM provides immunity to the host by building colonization resistance, a situation in which the innate GM antagonizes foreign microorganisms' colonization and prompts the preservation of structural and functional protective mucosal barriers [14, 15]. The GM in humans also invades and takeover foreign pathogens in the gut [19, 21]. The metabolites produced by GM, the short-chain fatty acids (SCFAs), reduces the intestinal pH, thus making survival difficult for foreign microorganisms [14, 15]. The functions of SCFAs will be discussed in subsequent sections of this chapter. In addition, the GM improves the integrity of intestinal mucosal to prevent invasion by foreign organisms. Another function of GM is the metabolism of xenobiotics [14, 15]. Xenobiotics, which are foreign materials to the bodies' biology, include drugs or chemicals that could be toxic [15]. Thus, the GM prevents the body from toxins by breaking them down from their harmful state.

2.2 The pathogenicity of the gut microbiota

Even though gut bacteria are beneficial, they could become pathogenic in their interaction with changes in the host environment and vectors. For example, if microorganisms giving benefits to the host invades other sites they do not usually colonize, that change in their environment could result in them acting as pathogens which could cause diseases [28, 29]. Furthermore, microorganisms in the body can also contribute to polymicrobial infections. Polymicrobial infection occurs when different microorganisms in the body interact and cooperate to create diseases in the host [28, 29]. Therefore, treatment has to be offered to take care of all microorganisms contributing to the infection.

One salient way the GM becomes harmful to the body is if its population in the gut undergoes unusual changes due to drug use, aging, sicknesses, lifestyle, and unhealthy food choices. This abnormal change in the population can result in gut dysbiosis (GD), which would be discussed in the subsequent section. In addition, changes to GM populations have been related to autoimmune situations, allergies, and chronic diseases. The incidence of diseases like autism, asthma, colitis, obesity, gestational diabetes, type 1 & 2 diabetes has been linked to GM's activity in its natural state or an altered nature [19]. Studies have equally shown a disparity in the types of GM or their populations present in a healthy and sick adult. For example, the type and population of GM in people living with gestational diabetes and type 2 diabetes differs from individuals free from the disease [24, 30]. The composition and population of the GM are identified to be influenced by factors such as diet, feeding type, birth delivery mode, and age of hosts [30, 31].

3. Phylum of gut bacteria in human body

Researchers identified the prominent type of GM colonizing the human gut, which is bacteria; therefore, subsequent sections of this chapter will focus on gut bacteria. Recently, scientists compiled data that shows there are about 2172 species of microorganisms isolated from humans. These species were classified into 12 phyla. The predominant phyla that make up about 93.5% of humans' colonies are bacteria, Proteobacteria, Actinobacteria, Bacteroidetes, and Firmicutes [13, 28]. Out of these four predominant phyla, 31·1% are phylum Firmicutes, particularly families Bacillaceae, 15.7%, and Clostridiaceae, 11·4% [28]. Proteobacteria occupies 29.5% of GM species isolated in humans, with 20% belonging to the family Enterobacteriaceae. Phylum Actinobacteria constitutes 25·9% of the GM isolated in humans, with 24·2% identifies as family Mycobacteriaceae. Bacteroidetes amount to 7·1% of the total species cultured from humans, and 29% of the phylum belongs to the family Prevotellaceae [15]. About 386 of the isolated species were identified to be anaerobic. Such microbiota would be found in the oral cavity and GIT – the mucosal regions [13].

3.1 Proteobacteria

Proteobacteria (PBAC) was initially called purple bacteria because of their reddish pigmentation, **Figure 2**. In 1988, a group of scientists studied the purple bacteria and their relatives. The scientists discovered that most of the bacteria and their relatives were neither purple nor photosynthetic. However, the bacteria group had great biological significance through physiological features. Therefore, scientists named these groups of microorganisms PBAC [31, 33, 34]. Characteristics of PBAC are:

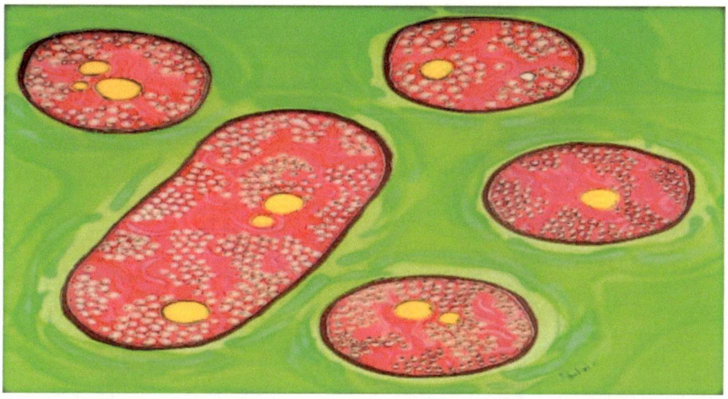

Figure 2.
Proteobacteria are called purple bacteria because of reddish pigmentation [32].

- The PBAC is gram-negative bacteria with an outer membrane made up of lipopolysaccharides. This outer membrane makes them resistant to drugs, particularly antibiotics [34, 35].

- The PBAC classes, families, and genera differ in motion and metabolic activities. They have different shapes. Some have flagella, some are non-motile, while some perform bacteria gliding [34, 35].

- The PBAC is facultative or obligatory anaerobic. They can be chemoautotrophs or heterotrophic, and they are pathogens [34, 35].

- Some classes and genera are of considerable importance to medical experts, food industries, and scientists within this phylum. Class Gammaproteobacteria includes important pathogens, *Salmonella*, *Vibrio*, *Pseudomonas*, *Escherichia*, *and Yersinia*. Genera such as *Helicobacter* and *Campylobacter* from class Epsilonproteobacteria are common in the GIT [34].

- Proteobacteria are allied to inflammation; therefore, their population increases in the gut in a condition prone to inflammation [31, 36].

3.2 Actinobacteria

Actinobacteria (ABAC), another populous bacteria in the human gut, are gram-negative bacteria and are mainly aerobic, even though some can survive under anaerobic conditions [37, 38]. The ABAC has other characteristics;

- The DNA of ABAC contains a high level of Guanine and Cytosine [37].

- Even though there are several genera, the pathogens that live in humans include Mycobacterium, Corynebacterium, Nocardia, and some species of Streptomyces [37, 38].

- The ABAC are secondary producers of metabolites; therefore, they are of interest for pharmacological and commercial purposes. The subclass Actinobacteridae and the order Actinomycetales are particularly of medical and economic benefit because their metabolites have antibiotics, particularly the genus Streptomyces [37, 38] (**Figure 3**).

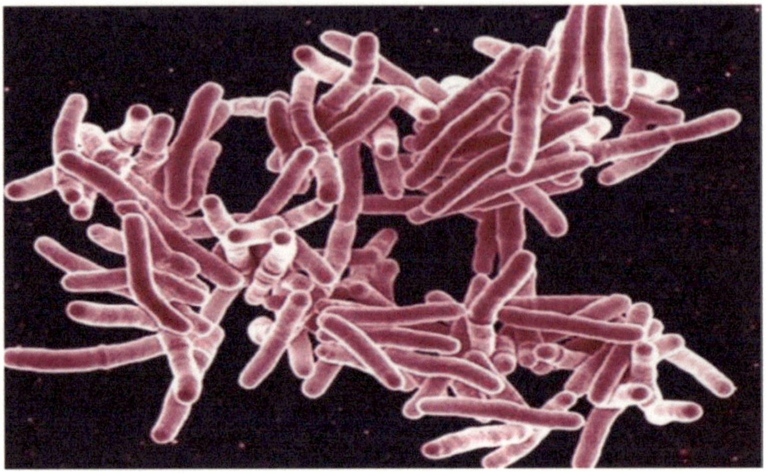

Figure 3.
Mycobacterium tuberculosis, *one of the species of Actinobacteria hosted by humans [39].*

3.3 Firmicutes

Firmicutes are gram-positive bacteria, though some have a pseudo outer membrane that makes them stain gram-negative [35, 40]. Phylum Firmicutes is notable for microorganisms that profer health benefits. Some genera of Firmicutes are administered as probiotics to profer gut health benefits. Characteristics include;

Firmicutes could be round (cocci) or rod-like (bacillus) in shape. Unlike the ABAC, they have a low level of Guanine and Cytosine in their DNA; they are acid-tolerant and take part in metabolic and physiological activities [35, 40].

There are two major classes; the anaerobic Clostridia and the obligate or facultative aerobic Bacilli [35, 40]. These are notable pathogens and beneficial microorganisms within this phylum. One crucial order of this phylum is the Lactobacillales (Lactic Acid Bacteria). Lactic acid bacteria produce lactic acid as a metabolite during glucose fermentation. Lactic Acid Bacteria appear everywhere in the food and are therefore regarded safe for consumption. In addition, they are known to contribute health benefits to the human gut [35, 40].

The genera for Lactic Acid Bacteria include *Lactococcus*, *Enterococcus*, and *Streptococcus*. The genus *Lactobacillus* (**Figure 4**) is the most common microbe used as probiotics [35, 40]. Firmicutes are either anaerobic, particularly *Clostridia*, while class Bacilli is an obligate or facultative aerobe. Therefore, bacteria belonging to class Bacilli would not grow or populate in an anaerobic environment [35, 40].

3.4 Bacteroidetes

Bacteroidetes are gram-negative, non-spore-forming, and anaerobic bacteria [42]. Bacteroidetes can survive in several environments, including the gut and skin. The class Bacteroidia is the most studied class of this phylum GM [42]. One common genus in this class is the *Bacteroides*. *Bacteroides* are clinically significant and have a mutualistic relationship with the host [42, 43]. The mutualistic behavior of *Bacteroides* occurs if they are retained in the gut. Once *Bacteroides* escape their familiar environment, they become pathogenic and can cause

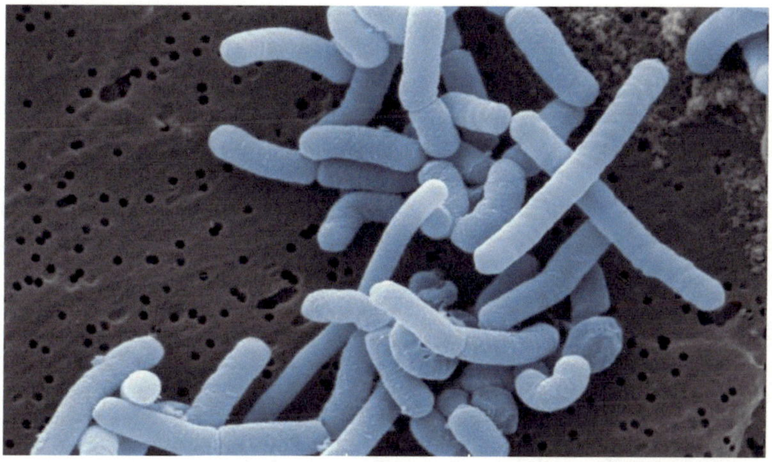

Figure 4.
Lactobacillus paracasei *[41].*

diseases such as an abscess in different parts of the body [43]. Other features of *Bacteroides* include:

- *Bacteroides* break down large molecules in the human guts into simpler molecules, while the bacteria derive their energy source from their host. The bacteria hence help to produce beneficial fatty acids [42, 43].

- *Bacteroides* prevent other pathogens from colonizing and infecting the gut of the host [42].

- *Bacteroides* have species that are highly resistant to many antibiotics [43]

4. Short-chain fatty acid producing bacteria

The GM is a balanced environment of different microorganisms such as bacteria, viruses, bacteriophages, archaea, and fungi; however, the bacteria community preserves the homeostasis of the gut. The bacteria community contains some groups of gut bacteria that produce SCFAs mentioned in Section 2.1.2. These fatty acids include acetate, propionate, and butyrate. The SCFAs are an essential fuel for the intestinal epithelial cells, and they assist the gut barrier functions and sustain homeostasis in the intestine [23, 44].

These groups of gut bacteria ferment indigestible dietary fibers to produce SCFAs. Dietary fibers such as resistant starch, inulin, wheat, oat bran, cellulose, pectin, and Guam gum are suitable substrates for bacteria activities and fermentation. Out of all prominent bacteria phylum identified in the human body, the Firmicutes and Bacteroidetes are more of the SCFAs producers [23, 44]. The acetate and propionate are produced by phylum Bacteroidetes, while the Firmicutes produce more of the butyrate [23, 45]. Another genus, such as *Bifidobacterium*, from phylum Actinobacteria and some Proteobacteria, could also produce butyrate. It is also important to note that some butyrate producers like Bacteroides are anaerobic bacteria and would not be active in aerobic situations; however, class Bacilli of Firmicutes would thrive because they are aerobes [23, 35, 46]. The aerobic environment in a human gut will suppress the growth of some butyrate-producing bacteria but allow the growth of aerobic pathogens like *Salmonella typhimurium* [23].

4.1 Functions of short-chain fatty acids in the gastrointestinal tract

1. The SCFAs control the gene expression for energy metabolism. Butyrate, in particular, is the primary energy source for colon cells. Therefore, SCFAs are involved in the energy metabolism of colon epithelial cells [23, 47, 48].

2. Propionate act as gluconeogenesis substrate in the intestine, where it can be oxidized to glucose. Acetate is also available in the tissues, where it can be transformed to butyrate and oxidized by muscles or used for lipogenesis [27, 49].

3. The SCFAs regulate the development of organoids. Hence, a cell proliferating attribute. The SCFA can induce mucus-secreting cells to secrete mucus that protects the mucosa [23, 48].

4. The SCFAs have been identified to suppress cancer cells or causing apoptosis to cancer cells. In addition, they perform the antimicrobial function because they can disrupt the osmotic and pH balance, creating an environment not accommodative to other microorganisms [48].

5. The SCFAs promote epithelial barrier function by initiating genes responsible for tight junctions and reforming protein, increasing epithelial resistance to pathogen invasion [23, 48].

6. The SCFAs induce prostaglandins which have an anti-inflammatory effect, thus reducing the pro-inflammatory effect. In addition, it induces anti-inflammatory cytokines to reduce the inflammation of the gut, which has been attributed to the cause of the host's susceptibility to some diseases [23, 49].

5. Interactions of gut microflora and diseases

The colonization of GM starts from childbirth; however, the composition starts changing based on different factors. For example, the birth delivery method, the mode of feeding, and the type of food offered to an infant determine GM's population [14, 22, 50]. For example, researchers reported that the type of bacteria composition in children fed with breast milk differs from children fed with the formula [14, 22]. In the same way, children born via natural birth have different GM compositions from children born via assisted delivery, such as caesarian surgery [14, 22]. As infants are introduced to solid food, GM composition makes another change [14, 22]. It is also important to note that the composition of GM also differs based on the part of GIT. For instance, the types of GM in the colon are different from the types in the stomach. This difference is because of factors such as the redox condition of the different organs. Other factors are the pH of the organ environment, allergies, the motility of organs, secretions in each organ such as the gastric acid secretion of the stomach, and the undamaged ileocaecal valve [14, 22]. Bacteria colonizing the guts from birth are also referred to as commensal bacteria because they benefit the host [14, 51]. For instance, Bacteroidetes and Firmicutes are the major phyla involved in breaking down macromolecules into simpler forms, particularly the indigestible fibers. However, abnormal changes can occur to the GM, leading to an abnormal composition of bacteria. This condition can be the onset of chronic diseases such as type 1 and 2 diabetes, obesity, cardiovascular diseases, cancer, and inflammatory bowel diseases [14, 52].

Surprisingly, abnormal bacteria composition has been linked with diseases that are considered temporary due to physiological changes like metabolic and immunological changes [7, 53]. An example is a gestational diabetes. During pregnancy, some women who cannot produce enough insulin develop gestational diabetes. The physiological changes occurring during pregnancy, such as weight gain, reduce the effective use of insulin, resulting in insulin resistance, as shown in **Figure 5**. The development of insulin resistance makes the body of the pregnant woman demands more insulin production. Even though gestational diabetes occurs late in pregnancy, some women experience insulin resistance before pregnancy [53, 55]. Women with gestational diabetes, if not well managed, might have their unborn babies at risk of being over 9lbs weight birth, which could bring delivery hazards to the mother. Also, the baby might be born earlier than anticipated, which could cause health problems for the baby. In addition, the baby might be born with low blood sugar. Women who have gestational diabetes are equally at a 40% risk of developing type 2 diabetes. About 5 to 20% of all world pregnancies are affected by gestational diabetes, and the percentage is increasing [7, 53, 56]. These statistics suggest a possible increase in people at risk of developing or living with type 2 diabetes, one of the world's major chronic diseases. Changes in the GM population are noticed in people who have gestational diabetes and chronic diseases. This change in population is the gut dysbiosis.

5.1 Gut dysbiosis

Gut dysbiosis is a condition in which there is a change in the balance of GM composition. Some phyla become highly populated while some reduce in population. This condition creates abnormality in the human GIT, and the pathogenesis of commensals bacteria starts [52]. Most bacteria in the gut are beneficial; however, when the balance in population changes in these bacteria gut colonies, as shown in **Figure 6**, dysbiosis occurs [7, 52]. Some symptoms of dysbiosis are mild and temporary; however, leaving dysbiosis untreated could result in severe symptoms associated with chronic diseases [52]. Even though commensals bacteria antagonize invading microorganisms, sometimes foreign microorganisms can seize the epithelium and overthrow the commensals, destabilizing the immune response [52]. After that, the invading pathogens induce inflammation to which they would be resistant, facilitating their growth and changing the balance of commensals bacteria. Viruses create series of mechanisms that regulate the activities of the

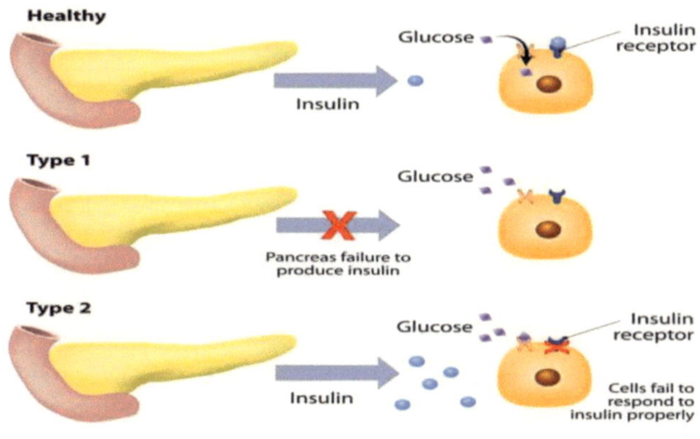

Figure 5.
Insulin resistance during gestational diabetes [54].

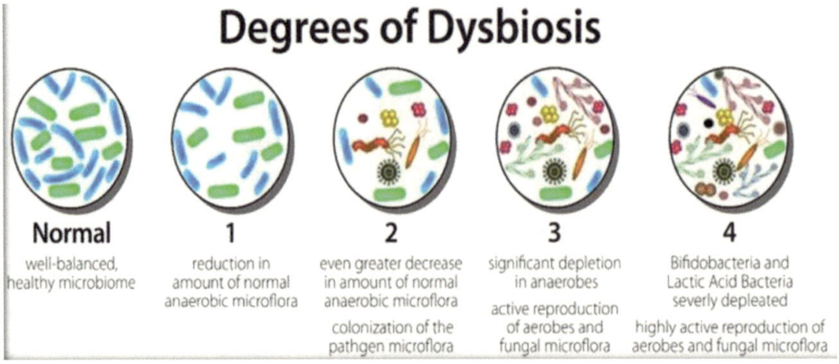

Figure 6.
Gut dysbiosis [57].

commensals, making them harmful to the host [16, 58]. Factors causing dysbiosis include a dietary change, chemical consumption like insecticides, alcoholism, improper use of medications, particularly antibiotics, poor dental hygiene, unprotected sex, stress, and anxiety, psychological stress. All these factors could change the balance of GM. In addition, the genotype and immune metabolic functions can alter the population of commensal microbes [52, 59, 60].

Symptoms of dysbiosis are dependent on the location of GM imbalance development and the types of bacteria involved. Symptoms could be gas, bloating, diarrhea, constipation, and cramps [52, 61]. To determine the imbalance of GM, most researchers make use of a human stool [52, 62]. The collected sample is then tested to determine the type of bacteria in the host's body. The organic acid test is another test used medically to determine imbalance [52, 62]. Some bacteria produce organic acids as metabolites. Therefore, the concentration of the organic acid in the urine sample determines the host's bacteria population. The hydrogen breath test is another test conducted to determine dysbiosis. In this case, gases from the mouth are tested for imbalance [52, 62]. Unfortunately, diseases tolerance varies in people; not everyone with dysbiosis shows severe symptoms that call for urgent attention or medical checkup, particularly at a young age. Ignoring or leaving the dysbiosis untreated, however, can result in many severe diseases.

5.2 Diseases associated with dysbiosis

The GM is partly responsible for the physiology of the body systems. Changes in the balance or population of GM have been linked to bowel diseases, allergies, and chronic metabolic diseases such as diabetes, obesity, cardiovascular diseases, and short-term disease like gestational diabetes.

5.2.1 Type 1 diabetes

According to research, Firmicutes such as *Lactobacillus*, Actinobacteria such as *Bifidobacterium* decreased in populations in children diagnosed with type 1 diabetes. In contrast, the population of Firmicutes such as *Clostridium* and *Veillonella*, Bacteroidetes like *Bacteroides* and *Prevotella* increased [14, 15]. Patients with Type 1 diabetes had low butyrate-producing and mucin degrading microbes, while pathogenic bacteria increased in population in the gut. Butyrate-producing bacteria and mucin degrading microbes are good for gut health [14, 63]. The functions of SCFAs, of which butyrate is one, are discussed in Section 4.1. Mucin degradation releases complex carbohydrates and produces SCFAs like acetate and propionate [64].

5.2.2 Type 2 diabetes

In patients with type 2 diabetes, Clostridia and Bacilli Firmicutes decreased in population while PBAC increased. Butyrate-producing microorganisms like Firmicutes are known to produce SCFAs. In addition, butyrate has the energy that provides 5–15% of the calories needed per individual daily [47, 65]. Therefore, Firmicutes' absence or reduced population in type 2 diabetes could elevate the blood glucose level. The increase in blood glucose is because the host will seek the missing calories by consuming more food. Lack or low butyrate concentration could also reduce satiety, making the host eat more, thus raising blood glucose [30, 47, 66].

Proteobacteria, which are more dominant in type 2 diabetes, induce inflammatory responses [36, 47]. An alteration in PBAC composition is common in metabolic syndromes causing diseases. In a study where the fecal samples of patients with type 2 diabetes were analyzed, a significant number of Enterobacteriaceae, a family from the phylum PBAC, were found [14, 31]. At the initiation of an inflammatory response, specific proteins are released into the bloodstream. These proteins inhibit insulin secretion and build insulin resistance in the body [14, 67].

5.2.3 Gestational diabetes

The profile of GM in women with gestational diabetes is similar to patients who have type 2 diabetes [53, 68]. In a study to determine the onset of dysbiosis in pregnant women, GM was typical in pregnant women in their first semester trimester. However, by the third trimester, the population of Proteobacteria and Actinobacteria increased while butyrate-producing microorganisms like *Faecalibacterium* and *Eubacterium* from phylum Firmicutes reduced. In addition, the Enterobacteriaceae family and *Streptococcus* were also numerous. Even though scientists observed Bacteroidetes and Firmicutes throughout all three trimesters of the pregnancy [68, 69]; however, the strong negative relationship between Bacteroidetes and Firmicutes phyla in healthy pregnant women was missing in women with gestational diabetes [7].

Most of the GM reduced were SCFA producing bacteria. The absence of these bacteria in pregnant women reduced the physiological function of the intestine. The gut permeability was not regulated, insulin sensitivity was reduced, inflammatory response that can lessen the development of diabetes was equally reduced [7]. Gut dysbiosis could be a biomarker for gestational diabetes, and a test of dysbiosis could be early detection before the pregnancy reaches the third trimester [7]. Changes in the GM population was associated with diet and weight gain during pregnancy [53, 68].

5.2.4 Inflammatory bowel disease

The two major bowel diseases associated with dysbiosis are Crohn's disease and ulcerative colitis [14, 15, 23]. In patients with Crohn's disease, the composition of GM was different from healthy individuals. Bacteria belonging to Firmicutes and Actinobacteria were decreased, some of which had a probiotic effect, while PBAC and *Ruminococcus gnavus*, another Firmicutes associated with inflammation, were increased [14, 24, 31, 70]. Increased susceptibility to Crohn's disease is attributed to a lack of the production of SCFAs. The PBAC is signaled as a pointer to instability in the microbiota. Therefore, an increase in the PBAC population is found in people with IBD disease. Even though the exact reason for the increase in PBAC is unknown, it is hypothesized that PBAC, with its inflammatory effect, creates anaerobic conditions in the gut. The beta-oxidation process reduces when proinflammation occurs. Therefore, anaerobic conditions contribute to the growth of PBAC, which are facultative anaerobe, thereby allowing dysbiosis [14, 15]. Anaerobic conditions increase the growth of pathogenic Firmicutes but reduce the population of the beneficial Firmicutes, like the Lactic Acid Bacteria [35, 40]. Another IBD due to dysbiosis is ulcerative colitis [14, 15]. Scientists discovered that *Lactobacilli* were low in composition in patients with ulcerative colitis at an active stage, while the Clostridiales order of Firmicutes was more prominent. High *Escherichia coli* was equally identified in people with active ulcerative colitis. Inflammation seen in IBD is associated with the decreased colonization resistance [14, 15].

Inflammatory Bowel Diseases (IBD) occur when genetic and environmental factors encourage the growth of pathogens that can decrease the population of commensals, thereby causing inflammation [15]. In addition, IBD can occur when there is an unusual immune response against commensal bacteria. For example, sometimes immune cells such as macrophages could not recognize GM and trigger an immune response which attacks the intestinal wall [15]. Hence, Firmicutes and Bacteroidetes decrease while PBAC increases.

5.2.5 Obesity

When the GM composition of healthy and patients with obesity were compared, anaerobic Firmicutes and Proteobacteria were increased in the fecal samples of patients. At the same time, Bacteroidetes decreased compared to a healthy individual. The high ratio of Firmicutes and Bacteroidetes has been linked to obesity [14, 71]. A significant increase in Enterobacteriaceae, PBAC family, was equally found in patients with obesity. This population of PBAC family reduced after the patient lost weight [31]. In a study on mice, a toll-like receptor 5, a sensor that detects microbial infection to initiate an immune response, was deficient when fed with a high-fat diet. The masking of toll-like receptor 5 concealed the changes occurring in the GM, and the body could not produce an immune response to fight the strange invading organisms [51, 72]. Deficiency of this receptor has been linked to hypertension, insulin resistance, and weight gain, though the exact reason for the masking was uncertain [15, 73].

5.2.6 Cardiovascular diseases

Microbiota dysbiosis was related to the development of cardiovascular diseases. A high level of PBAC was found in arteriosclerosis plaque, indicating PBAC has the pro-inflammatory effect that can cause plaque [15, 74]. In addition, some scientists reported that GM converts choline, an essential body nutrient, to trimethylamine, an organic compound. Trimethylamine is further processed in the liver to trimethylamine N-oxide which is known to increase arterial plaques. An increase in arterial plaque can cause arteriosclerosis diseases [14, 15]. In another study, Gammaproteobacteria, a class of PBAC, was connected with endogenous alcohol production linked to the cause of non-alcoholic fatty liver diseases, which is associated with increased risk of cardiovascular failure incidence [75].

5.2.7 Cancer

Inflammation caused by some phylum of GM could create a grave environment for the development and growth of cancer cells. Even though cancer linked to microbiota so far occurs in body parts that house the GM, notably the GIT, the colon [15, 76]. Commensals sometimes take up pathogenic features when invaded, giving them pathogenic effects; such commensals are called pathobionts. In a study on mice, pathobionts and pathogens contributed to the uncontrolled epithelial cell growth of the colorectal region [15]. Some scientists also suggested that some GM like *Bacillus fragilis*, a Bacteroidetes are virulent and can modify the GM to favor inflammatory responses. These inflammatory responses could cause alterations in the epithelial cells, and this could result in cancer. The inflammatory response will equally allow the invasion of cancer allies' microorganisms [15, 43]. In addition, people with chronic inflammatory disarray have been discovered to have a high susceptibility to gastric cancer and cancer of the lymphatic system associated with the mucosa [76].

6. Conclusion

Research continues on how GM and its activities cause chronic diseases. From completed studies, it is apparent that the composition of the gut differs between diseased and healthy individuals. While a significant population of commensals and SCFAs producing bacteria reduced, the pathogenic population increased and influenced the commensals, making them turn against the host. Pathogens equally created unfavorable conditions such as inflammatory or anaerobic conditions. The change in the environment favored the growth of pathogens but reduced the growth of commensals.

To take care of gut health, the types of food consumed determines the type of GM. Fermentable dietary fibers such as pectin, inulin, and resistant starch undergo fermentation by GM to produce 15% butyrate, 60% acetate, and 25% propionate. Butyrate maintains colonic homeostasis and prevents inflammation, and maintains mucosal integrity [44], thereby playing a role in reducing dysbiosis. Therefore, food rich in these fermentable dietary fibers would be suitable for gut health [25, 44]. The types of protein consumed matter to gut health. Animal protein fermentation decreases the production of SCFAs, increasing the risk of IBD [25]. However, consuming plant-based protein is associated with an increase in beneficial GM like *Bifidobacterium*, *Lactobacillus,* and it increases the production of SCFA [25, 44]. High consumption of polyunsaturated fatty acids has been associated with an increased healthy GM population like *Lactobacillus* and *Roseburia*, thus increasing the production of SCFA-butyrate [25, 44]. In contrast, high consumption of sodium and food additives such as sweeteners are associated with changes in the composition of GM. When food is high in sodium, it reduces the population of commensal microorganisms like *Lactobacillus*. Also, food additives cause a significant change in the population of the balanced gut system [25, 44]. What humans eat can determine gut health, and the composition of GM in the gut contributes to overall well-being.

Asides healthy diet, there are other ways to improve gut health. One of these ways is the use of probiotics as supplements. Probiotics are live microorganisms made into pills that profer health benefits when administered in adequate amounts. In addition, the use of prebiotics has equally been suggested. Prebiotics are not microorganisms but non-digestible substances that benefit the host by improving the growth and activities of selected bacteria in the gut [77–79]. Other methods are requiring medical experts and scientists. One is fecal microbiota transplantation, which involves infusing stool from a healthy donor to a recipient by delivering the stool through the upper GIT [80]. This method requires adequate care to ensure the feces transferred to other patients do not have infectious microorganisms. Other methods being used include phage therapy, bacteria consortium transplantation, and the use of predatory bacteria [81].

Acknowledgements

Special thanks to Olukayode Olubowale and Oluwaseun Sanusi for their contribution to the content of the chapter.

Author details

Temitope Sanusi-Olubowale[1,2]

1 Saybrook University, Oakland, California, USA

2 Albany State University, Albany, Georgia, USA

*Address all correspondence to: olutopy@gmail.com

References

[1] Centers for Disease Control and Prevention. About Chronic Diseases [Internet]. 2021. Available from https://www.cdc.gov/chronicdisease/about/index.htm [Accessed: 2021-04-19]

[2] Stoppler MC [Internet]. Medical Definition of Chronic disease. 2021. Available from https://www.medicinenet.com/chronic_disease/definition.htm [Accessed: 2021-07-10]

[3] World Health Organization. Integrated chronic disease prevention and control [Internet]. Available from https://www.who.int/chp/about/integrated_cd/en/ [Accessed: 2021-04-19]

[4] Barker DJ. Developmental origins of chronic disease. Public Health. 2012 Mar 1;126(3):185-9. DOI: https://doi.org/10.1016/j.puhe.2011.11.014

[5] Centers for Disease Control and Prevention. Health and Economic Costs of Chronic Diseases [Internet]. 2021. Available from https://www.cdc.gov/chronicdisease/about/costs/index.htm [Accessed 2021-04-19]

[6] Wilson PWF, D'Agostino RB, Levy D, Belanger AM, Silbershatz H, Kannel WB. Prediction of coronary heart disease using risk factor categories. Circulation. 1998 May 12;97(18):1837-47. DOI: https://doi.org/10.1161/01.CIR.97.18.1837

[7] Ma S, You Y, Huang L, Long S, Zhang J, Guo C, Zhang N, Wu X, Xiao Y, Tan H. Alterations in gut microbiota of gestational diabetes patients during the first trimester of pregnancy. Frontiers in cellular and infection microbiology. 2020 Feb 27;10:58. DOI: https://doi.org/10.3389/fcimb.2020.00058

[8] Baanders AN, Heijmans MJWM. The impact of chronic diseases: the partner's perspective. Family and Community Health. 2007;30:305-317. DOI: 10.1097/01.FCH.0000290543.48576.cf

[9] Bigatti SM, Cronan TA. An examination of the physical health, health care use, and psychological well-being of spouses of people with fibromyalgia syndrome. Health Psychology. 2002 Mar;21(2):157. DOI:10.1037/0278-6133.21.2.157

[10] Abegunde D, Stanciole A. An estimation of the economic impact of chronic noncommunicable diseases in selected countries. World Health Organization, Department of Chronic Diseases and Health Promotion. 2006; 2006. Available from https://www.who.int/chp/working_paper_growth%20model29may.pdf [Accessed: 2021-04-19]

[11] Milken Institute Study. Chronic disease costs US economy more than $1 trillion annually [Internet]. Available from https://www.fightchronicdisease.org/latest-news/milken-institute-study-chronic-disease-costs-us-economy-more-1-trillion-annually. [Accessed: 2021-07-10]

[12] Telford RD. Low physical activity and obesity: Causes of chronic disease or simply predictors? Medicine & Science in Sports & Exercise. 2007 Aug 1;39(8): 1233-40. DOI: 10.1249/mss.0b013e31806215b7

[13] Thursby E, Juge N. Introduction to the Human Gut Microbiota. Biochemical Journal. 2017;474(11):1823-1836. DOI: 10.1042/BCJ20160510

[14] Zhang YJ, Li S, Gan RY, Zhou T, Xu DP, Li HB. Impacts of gut bacteria on human health and diseases. International Journal of molecular sciences. 2015 Apr;16(4):7493-519. DOI: https://doi.org/10.3390/ijms16047493

[15] Blumberg R, Powrie F. Microbiota, disease, and back to health: a metastable journey. Science Translational Medicine. 2012 Jun 6;4(137):137rv7-. DOI: 10.1126/scitranslmed.3004184.

[16] Li N, Ma WT, Pang M, Fan QL, Hua JL. The commensal microbiota and viral infection: a comprehensive review. Frontiers in Immunology. 2019 Jul 4;10:1551. DOI: https://doi.org/10.3389/fimmu.2019.01551

[17] Looi M. The human microbiome: Everything you need to know about the 39 trillion microbes that call our bodies home [Internet]. 2020. Available from https://www.sciencefocus.com/the-human-body/human-microbiome/. [Accessed: 2021-07-10]

[18] National Institute of Health. NIH Human Microbiome Project defines normal bacterial makeup of the body: Genome sequencing creates first reference data for microbes living with healthy adults [Internet]. 2012. Available from https://www.nih.gov/news-events/news-releases/nih-human-microbiome-project-defines-normal-bacterial-makeup-body. [Accessed: 2021-07-10]

[19] McGill M. What are the gut microbiota and human microbiome? [Internet]. 2018. Available from https://www.medicalnewstoday.com/articles/307998 [Accessed 2021-04-19]

[20] Abbott A. Scientists bust myth that our bodies have more bacteria than human cells. Nature. 2016. DOI: https://doi.org/10.1038/nature.2016.19136

[21] Nuli R, Cai J, Kadeer A, Zhang Y, Patamu M. Integrative analysis toward different glucose tolerance-related gut microbiota and diet. Frontiers in Endocrinology. 2019;10(295):1-14. DOI: https://doi.org/10.3389/fendo.2019.00295

[22] Tanaka M, Nakayama J. Development of the gut microbiota in infancy and its impact on health in later life. Allergology International. 2017 Oct 1;66(4):515-22. DOI: https://doi.org/10.1016/j.alit.2017.07.010

[23] Parada VD, De la Fuente MK, Landskron G, González MJ, Quera R, Dijkstra G, Harmsen HJ, Faber KN, Hermoso MA. Short chain fatty acids (SCFAs)-mediated gut epithelial and immune regulation and its relevance for inflammatory bowel diseases. Frontiers in Immunology. 2019 Mar 11;10:277. DOI: https://doi.org/10.3389/fimmu.2019.00277

[24] Jandhyala SM, Talukdar R, Subramanyam C, Vuyyuru H, Sasikala M, Reddy DN. Role of the normal gut microbiota. World Journal of Gastroenterology. 2015; 21(29): 8787-8803. DOI: https://doi.org/10.3748/wjg.v21.i29.8787

[25] Robertson, R. 10 Ways to Improve Your Gut Bacteria, Based on Science [Internet]. 2016. Available from https://www.healthline.com/nutrition/improve-gut-bacteria. [Accessed: 2021-06-27]

[26] Kieffer DA, Martin RJ, Adams SH. Impact of dietary fibers on nutrient management and detoxification organs: Gut, liver, and kidneys. Advances in Nutrition. 2016 Nov 15;7(6):1111-1121. DOI: 10.3945/an.116.013219.

[27] De Vadder F, Kovatcheva-Datchary P, Goncalves D, Vinera J, Zitoun C, Duchampt A, Backhed F, Mithieux G. Microbiota-generated metabolites promote metabolic benefits via gut-brain neural circuits. Cell. 2014 Jan 16;156(1-2):84-96. DOI: https://doi.org/10.1016/j.cell.2013.12.016

[28] Hugon P, Dufour J, Colson P, Fournier P, Sallah K, Raoult D. A comprehensive repertoire of prokaryotic species identified in human beings. The Lancet Infectious Diseases. 2015 10;15(10):1211-1219. DOI:10.1016/S1473-3099(15)00293-5

[29] Brogden KA, Guthmiller JM, Taylor CE. Human polymicrobial infections. Lancet. 2005 Jan 15-21;365(9455):253-5. DOI: 10.1016/S0140-6736(05)17745-9

[30] Gerard C, Vidal H. Impact of gut microbiota on host glycemic control.

Frontiers in Endocrinology. 2019;10(29): 1-13. DOI: https://doi.org/10.3389/fendo.2019.00029

[31] Rizzatti G, Lopetuso LR, Gibiino G, Binda C, Gasbarrini A. Proteobacteria: A common factor in human diseases. BioMed Research International. 2017 Oct;2017. DOI: https://doi.org/10.1155/2017/9351507

[32] Noel O. Purple bacteria or purple photosynthetic bacteria are pigmented by bacteriochlorophyll and carotenoids, giving them a colorful range of purples, pinks and oranges. They photosynthesize without producing oxygen as a by-product. This type of bacteria are proteobacteria which are phototrophic (produce their own food via photo-synthesis). [Internet]. Available from https://wellcomecollection.org/works/zermwrgw [Accessed: 2021-07-03]

[33] Stackebrandt E, Murray RG, Truper HG. Proteobacteria classis nov., A name for the phylogenetic taxon that includes the "purple bacteria and their relatives." International Journal of Systematic and Evolutionary Micro-biology. 1988 Jul 1;38(3):321-5. DOI: https://doi.org/10.1099/00207713-38-3-321

[34] Overview of Proteobacteria [Internet]. 2021. Available from: https://bio.libretexts.org/@go/page/9775 [Accessed 2021-04-19]

[35] Encyclopedia of life. Purple bacteria and relatives [Internet]. Available from https://eol.org/pages/311/articles Accessed: 2021-07-09

[36] Satokari R. High intake of sugar and the balance between pro-and anti-inflammatory gut bacteria. Nutrients. 2020;12(5):1-4. DOI: https://doi.org/10.3390/nu12051348

[37] Actinobacteria (High G + C Gram-Positive Bacteria) [Internet]. 2021. Available from: https://bio.libretexts.org/@go/page/9786 [Accessed 2021-04-19]

[38] Anandan R, Dharumadurai D, Manogaran GP. An Introduction to Actinobacteria. In Dharumadurai D, Jiang Y, editors. Actinobacteria - Basics and Biotechnological Applications. Intechopen; 2016. DOI: 10.5772/62329

[39] National Institute of Allergy and Infectious Diseases (NIAID). *Mycobacterium tuberculosis* Bacteria, the cause of TB. Available from https://www.flickr.com/photos/54591706@N02/5149398656 [Accessed: 2021-7-7]

[40] Firmicutes [Internet]. 2021. Available from: https://bio.libretexts.org/@go/page/978 [Accessed 2021-04-19]

[41] Neve H, Rubner M. "File: *Lactobacillus paracasei*.jpg" 2018. Available from https://search.creativecommons.org/photos/728ca0ee-110a-4b06-b639-60444e0a801d [Accessed: 2021-07-07]

[42] Bacteroidetes and Chlorobi [Internet]. 2021. Available from: https://bio.libretexts.org/@go/page/9799 [Accessed 2021-04-19]

[43] Wexler HM. Bacteroides: the good, the bad, and the nitty-gritty. Clinical Microbiology Reviews. 2007 Oct;20(4): 593-621. DOI: 10.1128/CMR.00008-07

[44] Rinninella E, Cintoni M, Raoul P, Lopetuso LR, Scaldaferri F, Pulcini G, Miggiano GA, Gasbarrini A, Mele MC. Food components and dietary habits: Keys for a healthy gut microbiota composition. Nutrients. 2019 Oct; 11(10):2393. DOI: 10.3390/nu11102393

[45] Chakraborti CK. New-found link between microbiota and obesity. World journal of gastrointestinal pathophysiology. 2015 Nov 15;6(4):110. DOI: 10.4291/wjgp.v6.i4.110

[46] Bai Y, Mansell TJ. Production and Sensing of Butyrate in a Probiotic *E. coli*

Strain. International Journal of molecular sciences. 2020 Jan;21(10):3615. DOI: 10.3390/ijms21103615

[47] Stewart L. What is butyrate and why should you care? [Internet]. Atlas. 2021. Available from https://atlasbiomed.com/blog/what-is-butyrate/ [Accessed 2021-04-28]

[48] Tan J, McKenzie C, Potamitis M, Thorburn AN, Mackay CR, Macia L. The role of short-chain fatty acids in health and disease. Advances in Immunology. 2014 Jan 1;121:91-119. DOI: https://doi.org/10.1016/B978-0-12-800100-4.00003-9

[49] Chambers ES, Preston T, Frost G, Morrison DJ. Role of gut microbiota-generated short-chain fatty acids in metabolic and cardiovascular health. Current Nutrition Reports. 2018 Dec;7(4):198-206.

[50] Backhed F, Roswall J, Peng Y, Feng Q, Jia H, Kovatcheva-Datchary P, Li Y, Xia Y, Xie H, Zhong H, Khan MT. Dynamics and stabilization of the human gut microbiome during the first year of life. Cell Host & Microbe. 2015 May 13;17(5):690-703. DOI: https://doi.org/10.1016/j.chom.2015.04.004

[51] Khan R, Petersen FC, Shekhar S. Commensal bacteria: An emerging player in defense against respiratory pathogens. Frontiers in Immunology. 2019 May 31;10:1203. DOI: 10.3389/fimmu.2019.01203.

[52] Jewell T. What Causes Dysbiosis and How Is It Treated? [Internet]. 2019. Available from https://www.healthline.com/health/digestive-health/dysbiosis [Accessed 2021-04-28]

[53] Crusell MK, Hansen TH, Nielsen T, Allin KH, Ruhlemann MC, Damm P, Vestergaard H, Rorbye C, Jorgensen NR, Christiansen OB, Heinsen FA. Gestational diabetes is associated with change in the gut microbiota composition in third trimester of pregnancy and postpartum. Microbiome. 2018 Dec;6(1):1-9. DOI: https://doi.org/10.1186/s40168-018-0472-x

[54] Dereke J. Gestational diabetes: A novel detection strategy [Internet]. Research Outreach. 2019. Available from: https://researchoutreach.org/articles/gestational-diabetes-novel-detection-strategy/ DOI: 10.32907/RO-110-148151

[55] Centers for Disease Control and Prevention. Gestational Diabetes [Internet]. 2019. Available from https://www.cdc.gov/diabetes/basics/gestational.html [Accessed 2021-07-01]

[56] Behboudi-Gandevani S, Amiri M, Yarandi RB, Tehrani FR. The impact of diagnostic criteria for gestational diabetes on its prevalence: A systematic review and meta-analysis. Diabetology & Metabolic Syndrome. 2019 Dec;11(1):1-8. DOI: https://doi.org/10.1186/s13098-019-0406-1

[57] Biospec Nutritionals. Gut health and gastrointestinal (GI) imbalances. Available from https://biospec-nutritionals.com/health-topics/gut-health-and-gastrointestinal-gi-imbalances/. [Accessed: 2021-04-28]

[58] Karst SM. The influence of commensal bacteria on infection with enteric viruses. Nature Reviews Microbiology. 2016;14:197-204. DOI: 10.1038/nrmicro.2015.25

[59] Biospec Nutritionals. Gut health and gastrointestinal (GI) imbalances. Available from https://biospec nutritionals.com/health-topics/gut-health-and-gastrointestinal-gi-imbalances/. [Accessed: 2021-04-28].

[60] Myers SP, Hawrelak JA. The causes of intestinal dysbiosis: a review. Alternative Medicine Review. 2004 Jun;9(2):180-97. Available from https://altmedrev.com/wp-content/uploads/2019/02/v9-2-180.pdf [Accessed: 2021-4-30]

[61] Atlas. Microbiome Testing: What Is Dysbiosis And Do You Check For It? Available from https://atlasbiomed.com/blog/dysbiosis-and-microbiome-testing/ [Accessed 2021-06-13]

[62] Laguipo ABB. Dysbiosis Diagnosis. 2018. [Internet] Available from https://www.news-medical.net/health/Dysbiosis-Diagnosis.aspx [Accessed: 2021-07-10]

[63] Vaarala O. Human intestinal microbiota and type 1 diabetes. Current Diabetes Reports. 2013 Oct 1;13(5):601-7. DOI:10.1007/s11892-013-0409-5

[64] Van Herreweghen F, De Paepe K, Roume H, Kerckhof FM, Van de Wiele T. Mucin degradation niche as a driver of microbiome composition and *Akkermansia muciniphila* abundance in a dynamic gut model is donor independent. FEMS microbiology ecology. 2018 Dec;94(12):fiy186. DOI: https://doi.org/10.1093/femsec/fiy186

[65] Larsen N, Vogensen FK, van den Berg FW, Nielsen DS, Andreasen AS, Pedersen BK, Al-Soud WA, Sørensen SJ, Hansen LH, Jakobsen M. Gut microbiota in human adults with type 2 diabetes differs from non-diabetic adults. PLoS One. 2010 Feb 5;5(2):e9085. DOI: 10.1371/journal.pone.0009085.

[66] Dickson I. Intestinal gluconeogenesis prevents hepatic steatosis. Nature Review Gastroenterology Hepatology. 2020;17: 316. DOI: https://doi.org/10.1038/s41575-020-0301-0

[67] Rehman K, Akash MSH. Mechanisms of inflammatory responses and development of insulin resistance: How are they interlinked? Journal of Biomedical Science. 2016;23(87):1-18. DOI: https://doi.org/10.1186/s12929-016-0303-y

[68] Hasain Z, Mokhtar NM, Kamaruddin NA, Mohamed Ismail NA, Razalli NH, Gnanou JV, Raja Ali RA. Gut microbiota and gestational diabetes mellitus: A review of host-gut microbiota interactions and their therapeutic potential. Frontiers in Cellular and Infection Microbiology. 2020 May 15;10:188. DOI: https://doi.org/10.3389/fcimb.2020.00188

[69] Koren O, Goodrich JK, Cullender TC, Spor A, Laitinen K, Bäckhed HK, Gonzalez A, Werner JJ, Angenent LT, Knight R, Bäckhed F. Host remodeling of the gut microbiome and metabolic changes during pregnancy. Cell. 2012 Aug 3;150(3):470-80. DOI: 10.1016/j.cell.2012.07.008

[70] Henke MT, Kenny DJ, Cassilly CD, Vlamakis H, Xavier RJ, Clardy J. Ruminococcus gnavus, a member of the human gut microbiome associated with Crohn's disease, produces an inflammatory polysaccharide. Proceedings of the National Academy of Sciences. 2019 Jun 25;116(26):12672-7. DOI: https://doi.org/10.1073/pnas.1904099116

[71] Gerard P. Gut microbiota and obesity. Cellular and Molecular Life Sciences. 2016 Jan 1;73(1):147-62. DOI 10.1007/s00018-015-2061-5

[72] Feuillet V, Medjane S, Mondor I, Demaria O, Pagni PP, Galán JE, Flavell RA, Alexopoulou L. Involvement of Toll-like receptor 5 in the recognition of flagellated bacteria. Proceedings of the National Academy of Sciences. 2006 Aug 15;103(33):12487-92. DOI: https://doi.org/10.1073/pnas.0605200103

[73] Vijay-Kumar M, Aitken JD, Carvalho FA, Cullender TC, Mwangi S, Srinivasan S, Sitaraman SV, Knight R, Ley RE, Gewirtz AT. Metabolic syndrome and altered gut microbiota in mice lacking Toll-like receptor 5. Science. 2010;328:228-231.

[74] Wang Z, Klipfell E, Bennett BJ, Koeth R, Levison BS, Dugar B, Feldstein AE, Britt EB, Fu X, Chung YM, Wu Y, Schauer P, Smith JD,

Allayee H, Tang WH, DiDonato JA, Lusis AJ, Hazen SL. Gut flora metabolism of phosphatidylcholine promotes cardiovascular disease. Nature. 2011;472:57-63. DOI: 10.1038/nature09922

[75] Tana C, Ballestri S, Ricci F, Di Vincenzo A, Ticinesi A, Gallina S, Giamberardino MA, Cipollone F, Sutton R, Vettor R, Fedorowski A. Cardiovascular risk in non-alcoholic fatty liver disease: Mechanisms and therapeutic implications. International Journal of Environmental Research and Public Health. 2019 Jan;16(17):3104. DOI: 10.3390/ijerph16173104

[76] Cheng WY, Wu C, Yu J. The role of gut microbiota in cancer treatment: Friend or foe? Gut. 2020;69:1867-1876 DOI:http://dx.doi.org/10.1136/gutjnl-2020-321153

[77] Dix M. What's an unhealthy gut? How gut health affects you [Internet]. 2020. Available from https://www.healthline.com/health/gut-health. Accessed: 2021-07-15]

[78] Nutrition Division. Health and nutritional properties of probiotics in food, including powder milk with live lactic acid bacteria. FAO Food and Nutrition Paper. 2006;85. Available from http://www.fao.org/3/a0512e/a0512e.pdf. [Accessed: 2021-07-15]

[79] Gibson GR, Roberfroid MB. Dietary modulation of the human colonic microbiota: introducing the concept of prebiotics. The Journal of nutrition. 1995 Jun 1;125(6):1401-12. DOI: https://doi.org/10.1093/jn/125.6.1401

[80] Kim KO, Gluck M. Fecal microbiota transplantation: an update on clinical practice. Clinical endoscopy. 2019 Mar;52(2):137. DOI: 10.5946/ce.2019.009

[81] Gagliardi A, Totino V, Cacciotti F, Iebba V, Neroni B, Bonfiglio G, Trancassini M, Passariello C, Pantanella F, Schippa S. Rebuilding the gut microbiota ecosystem. International journal of environmental research and public health. 2018 Aug;15(8):1679. DOI: https://doi.org/10.3390/ijerph15081679

Section 2

Management of Gestational Diabetes Mellitus

Chapter 4

Improving Gestational Diabetes Management through Patient Education

Radiana Staynova and Vesselina Yanachkova

Abstract

The challenge of achieving a healthy pregnancy and a successful birth outcome in women with gestational diabetes mellitus (GDM) requires a multidisciplinary approach with close collaboration between healthcare providers. One of the key elements for the successful management of GDM is the education of pregnant women. Patient education has been shown to improve quality of life, contribute to better compliance, and reduce complications and healthcare costs. In this chapter, we will present and discuss the main barriers in the educational process of women with GDM and innovative approaches for improving diabetes self-management education during pregnancy. The focus will be on the different educational methods, such as printed leaflets and booklets, Web-based educational programs, and new technologies including telemedicine and smartphone applications.

Keywords: gestational diabetes, patient education, pregnancy, booklet, telemedicine

1. Introduction

Pregnancy is a specific condition that is associated with significant changes in the course of metabolic processes in the female body [1]. Gestational diabetes mellitus (GDM) is a common pregnancy complication and it was estimated that it affects 1 in 6 births [2]. GDM is associated with multiple adverse pregnancy outcomes including caesarian delivery, preeclampsia, subsequent development of type 2 diabetes, macrosomia, shoulder dystocia, neonatal hypoglycemia, and respiratory distress syndrome [3].

GDM can be a scary experience in the beginning, and it can take time for a pregnant woman to make the necessary changes to ensure optimal control. In addition to the potential risks it poses to the mother and fetus, GDM can also have a negative effect on the mental health and quality of life of pregnant women [4, 5].

In most cases, GDM is a temporary condition that usually occurs between 24 and 28 weeks of gestation and disappears after a woman gives birth. However, its occurrence poses a risk in affected women for the development of type 2 diabetes in the future [6]. There are no generally accepted standards for diagnosing GDM, which is why many women do not receive the treatment they need to achieve successful birth outcomes [7].

Women diagnosed with GDM need detailed information and appropriate education on the pathophysiology of GDM, treatment options, self-management (self-monitoring of blood glucose, meal planning, exercise), and possible complications of this condition [8]. Education is the key element in the diabetes care process. It provides an opportunity for women with GDM to realize their place and role in the diabetes team. The main education strategy during pregnancy is aimed at acquiring knowledge and skills for adaptation and self-management of diabetes [9].

Providing education and counseling to women with GDM can sometimes face additional challenges and barriers [8]. For improving diabetes self-management education during pregnancy and overcome these challenges, innovative approaches can be used.

2. Diabetes education during pregnancy

Dr. Elliott P. Joslin (1869–1962) is considered to be the founder of modern diabetes education. As early as 1925, he conducted educational courses that included an explanation of the disease, insulin treatment, food intake, and physical activity. Dr. Joslin is also the author of the first diabetes patient handbook called "Diabetic Manual—for the Doctor and Patient" [10]. Part of the Joslin Clinic team was Dr. Priscilla White (1900–1989), who is considered a pioneer in the treatment of diabetes during pregnancy [11].

Pregnancy complicated by diabetes can be an adventure full of challenges. During this adventure, pregnant women require additional information, education, support, as well as appropriate treatment and practical advice for self-management. All this requires the active involvement of the woman with GDM, her family, and the diabetes team. Newly diagnosed women sometimes feel scared and insecure about how they will deal with GDM self-management. Providing structured education, support, and trust-building partnership between the patient and a well-collaborating diabetes team is crucial to acquiring knowledge and skills in managing the "sweet" disease [12]. According to Okun et al., an effective healthcare partnership includes health providers working in concert with patients and family caregivers to achieve positive experience and mutually agreed-upon outcomes [13].

Providing diabetes education is a keystone in a comprehensive therapeutic approach. Patients should gain knowledge, skills, and motivation to overcome daily challenges associated with the disease [9, 14]. Diabetes self-management education in parallel with insulin discovery is considered to be one of the most important advances in diabetes treatment in the 20th century [9].

The education of women with GDM is very important for the normal course of pregnancy and avoidance of complications. If a woman has not had diabetes before pregnancy, she may not know how to measure and track her blood glucose levels or how to administer insulin.

The main goals of the education process of women with GDM include the following:

- Optimization of knowledge about diabetes pathophysiology, risk factors, and management;
- Increasing the pregnant women's motivation to take care of themselves;
- Effective compliance with diet and performing physical activity;
- Meal planning and carbohydrate counting;

- Instructions for administrating insulin and recommendations for dealing with side effects (e.g., hypoglycemia);

- Self-monitoring and tracking of blood glucose levels;

- Effective communication between members of the diabetes team;

- Prevention of type 2 diabetes later in life.

In 2017, International Diabetes Federation (IDF) developed interactive online courses called the IDF School of Diabetes. These educational programs consist of several modules that cover all aspects of diabetic care, disease management, and prevention. The courses are certified and end with a final exam. They are suitable for all health professionals involved in diabetes care, including general practitioners, nurses, pharmacists, dietitians, social workers, and others. In addition to training, the Web site also offers access to information on the latest advances in diabetes therapy. The main mission of the IDF School of Diabetes is to provide innovative educational programs for health professionals involved in the care and treatment of diabetes, which in turn provide the necessary training resources to people with diabetes and those who care for them [15].

In Bulgaria, in 1997, a unified large-scale training program for patients with diabetes was introduced, supported by the Government of Denmark and the Bulgarian Ministry of Health. There are 56 training centers in the country—4 university centers, 48 regional centers, and 4 training centers for children with diabetes, in which a structured five-day training program for patients has been introduced. Initially, teams of doctors and nurses from the Medical Universities of Sofia, Plovdiv, Varna,

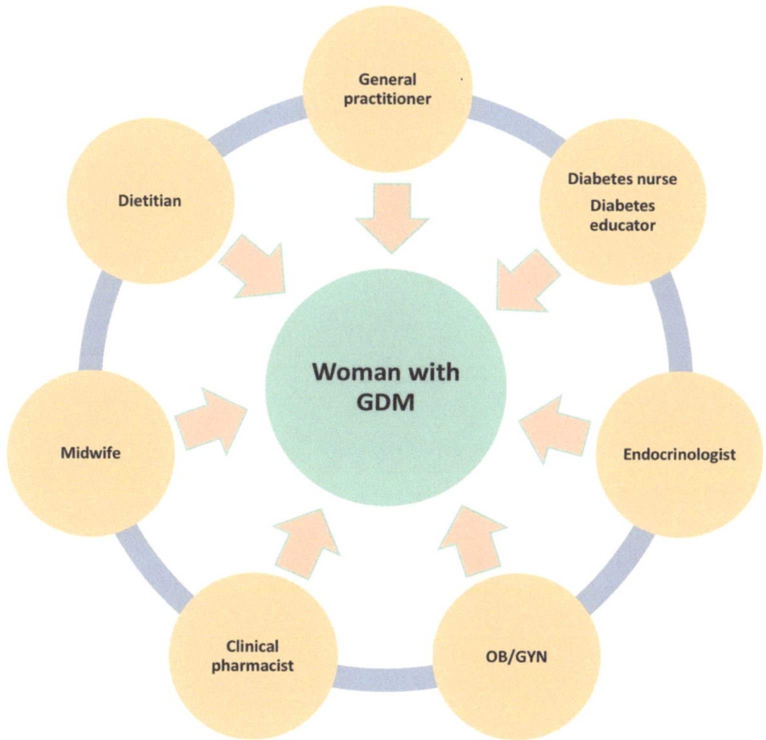

Figure 1.
The diabetes team involved in the educational process of woman with GDM.

and Pleven were trained at the Steno Diabetes Center in Copenhagen, after which they organized the training of other teams in the country [16].

The challenge of achieving a healthy pregnancy and a successful birth outcome in women with GDM requires a multidisciplinary approach with close collaboration between healthcare providers. The diabetes team involved in the educational process may include medical professionals with different specialties (**Figure 1**).

The education for women with GDM focuses on their needs, preferences, and goals, helping to increase not only the knowledge about the disease but also to provide skills related to self-management and treatment [17]. Patient education has been shown to improve quality of life, contribute to better compliance, and reduce complications and healthcare costs [17–20].

3. Barriers in the educational process of women with GDM

In the educational process, the diabetes team often encounters difficulties of different nature, which may affect both healthcare providers and pregnant women [14]. These difficulties or barriers could be classified as patient-related, healthcare provider-related, and socioeconomic or cultural barriers (**Figure 2**).

The most common barriers related to pregnant women include lack of motivation, inpatient behavior, low level of trust in healthcare providers, poor adherence and compliance to health advice, a tendency to deny their own role in the process of education, or not being willing to assist in the implementation of instructions and prescriptions. There may also be barriers related to healthcare providers such as the use of a non-motivational approach, poor communication skills, insufficient time, lack of special qualifications. Other barriers that may

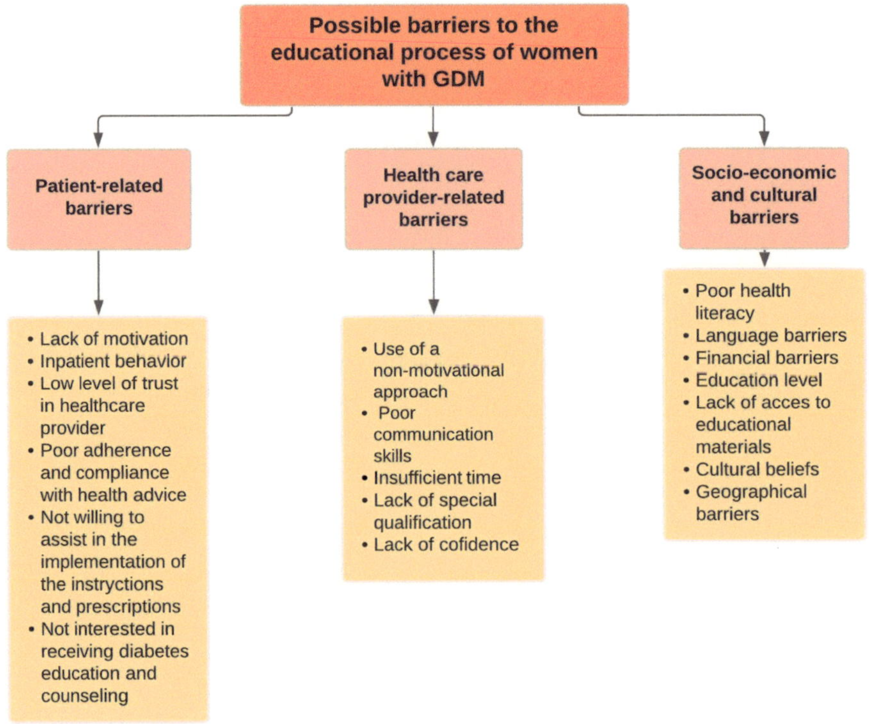

Figure 2.
Possible barriers to the educational process of women with GDM.

occur during the education process include socioeconomic factors, geographical factors, cultural factors, level of education of patients, poor health literacy, and lack of access to educational materials [14].

Different strategies could be used for overcoming barriers during the educational process. These strategies may include demonstrations, written information (leaflets, brochures, booklets, etc.), pictograms, audio and video materials, and mobile applications.

4. Printed leaflets and booklets

Verbal or oral communication is essential for the educational process, but it is not enough in itself. The provision of printed educational materials such as leaflets and booklets in addition to healthcare provider counseling makes patient education more effective [21]. The use of written informational materials in the educational process can improve the quality of life, contribute to better compliance, prevent complications, and reduce healthcare costs [22].

Printed leaflets and booklets must meet the basic requirements for the effectiveness of the written educational materials in terms of content, structure, language, layout, and illustrations [22]. Using plain language, followed by appropriate charts, figures, and illustrations, is essential in the development process of printed educational materials [23]. The information included in them must be based on reliable, publicly available, and evidence-based literature sources. Attractive visualization is very important for a better understanding of the information included in the leaflets/booklets [22, 24]. Printed educational materials should provide practical and easy-to-follow advice to help pregnant women manage their condition successfully.

Some of the diabetes associations and health organizations have developed informational brochures and guidelines designed especially for women with GDM. IDF has developed an educational manual entitled "Having a baby? Now is the time to learn more about gestational diabetes?" which aims to provide information about GDM in an easy-to-understand form for expectant mothers [25]. American Diabetes Association provides information on GDM on its Web site, as well as in the book "Pregnancy & Diabetes: A Complete Guide for Women with Gestational, Type 2, And Type 1 Diabetes" [26]. In the USA, The Centers for Disease Control and Prevention also provides a brochure about GDM and pregnancy [27]. In Australia, National Diabetes Services Scheme developed an educational booklet that provides comprehensive information on GDM management and where pregnant women can get additional help. In addition to the English version, the brochure is also available in seven other languages [28].

In Bulgaria, we developed an educational manual for healthy pregnancy designed for women with GDM [29]. The educational manual gives the readers realistic insight and practical advice on how to deal with the daily challenges of pregnancy with diabetes. It covers all the aspects of GDM management (medical nutrition therapy; recipes for healthy meals; exercise tips for pregnancy: types, benefits, and cautions; insulin use; self-monitoring of blood glucose; sources of additional information and support—mobile applications, technologies, and Web sites). Information about the follow-up of GDM and prevention of type 2 diabetes has also been included. A feedback study showed a very high level of patient satisfaction. Pregnant women find the educational manual very useful [30].

Even in the modern digital age, written health information could play an important role in improving the connection between the patient and the healthcare provider. The provision of printed educational materials can increase patients' health literacy, as well as their personal responsibility, motivation, and attitude toward their own health. The development of printed educational materials about GDM may improve pregnant women's knowledge, their lifestyle habits (appropriate weight gain, meal planning, physical activity, etc.), and regular self-monitoring of blood glucose (four times daily), and contribute to avoiding maternal and fetal complications.

5. Telemedicine and Web-based education

Telemedicine can be defined as a way of providing medical services remotely without physical contact between the healthcare provider and the patient, most often through a telephone conversation or video link through a platform [31]. The rapid development of digital technologies in recent years has turned telemedicine into an important component of healthcare delivery [32]. During the COVID-19 pandemic, telemedicine allowed patients to communicate completely safely and effectively with their healthcare providers [33]. Diabetes care is the area where telemedicine finds wide application [34].

A recent systematic review evaluated the effectiveness of telemedicine interventions for women with GDM. The meta-analysis included 32 randomized controlled trials and showed that telemedicine was associated with significant improvement in glycemic control (HbA1c, fasting, and postprandial blood glucose levels) and lower incidence of adverse pregnancy outcomes (Cesarean sections, neonatal hypoglycemia, macrosomia, preterm birth) compared to standard care [35].

The use of telemedicine in the management of GDM may have notable benefits. More cost evaluation studies are required to confirm its cost-effectiveness.

Since the Internet is found to be the primary source of information during pregnancy, the use of Web-based education programs for women with GDM could have a beneficial effect on diabetes self-management [36]. In Australia, Carolan et al. developed and tested an educational Web site for women with GDM [37]. The researchers assessed pregnant women's knowledge of GDM and healthy lifestyle (healthy diet and foods), after using the Web-based program compared to women who received standard education. The findings showed that both approaches resulted in excellent knowledge scores [36]. Recent randomized control trial (RCT) using the same Web site aimed to evaluate changes in maternal body mass index, blood pressure, glycemic level, and infant birth weight after using a Web-based educational program compared to standard clinic-based GDM education. Results showed significant improvements in the intervention group that received Web-based education. Significant differences were observed between groups regarding women's postpartum weight, glycemic level, and attendance at oral glucose tolerance test by 12-week postpartum [38].

6. Smartphone applications

In today's digital age, in addition to the role of medical professionals who care for women with GDM, a new assistant would take part: mobile applications.

There are mobile applications (apps) designed specifically for women with GDM, which are already popular and highly desired among pregnant women [39, 40].

A recent study performed by Zahmatkeshan et al. aimed to review the evidence for the effectiveness of using mobile health (m-health) interventions for GDM. Based on their findings, it can be concluded that m-health interventions, including apps, could have a positive effect on GDM management and outcomes [41].

Another study evaluated the mobile apps applicability for pregnant women at risk of GDM. According to the results, the authors suggest that there is a need for the development of more apps that provide both comprehensive educational content and tracking tools [42].

There are few RCTs that assess the effects of mobile apps on GDM management [39, 43–46]. The largest one [46] was conducted in Singapore among 340 pregnant women with GDM. The results from this study show that in addition to usual care, the use of a smartphone app coaching program led to better glycemic control and fewer neonatal complications [46].

Mobile apps cannot replace consulting a healthcare provider, but they could be useful in GDM management.

7. Conclusion

This chapter summarizes all of the aspects of diabetes self-management education during pregnancy including possible challenges and innovative approaches that can find practical application in the educational process. Health professionals can encourage women with GDM to look for mobile apps, Web sites, and new technologies that can help them to successfully manage the disease. Active involvement of pregnant women and good collaboration of the diabetes team member is essential for the effectiveness of the educational process.

Acknowledgements

The publication of this chapter was financially funded by Novo Nordisk. The authors take full responsibility for the content and conclusions stated in this manuscript. Novo Nordisk neither influenced the content of this publication nor was it involved in the study design, data collection, analysis, interpretation or review.

Conflict of interest

The authors declare no conflict of interest.

Author details

Radiana Staynova[1]* and Vesselina Yanachkova[2]

1 Faculty of Pharmacy, Department of Pharmaceutical Sciences, Medical University of Plovdiv, Plovdiv, Bulgaria

2 Department of Endocrinology, Specialized Hospital for Active Treatment of Obstetrics and Gynecology "Dr. Shterev", Sofia, Bulgaria

*Address all correspondence to: radiana.staynova@mu-plovdiv.bg

References

[1] Ianatchkova V, Chaveeva P, Shterev A. The gestational diabetes mellitus as a specific pregnancy state. Akush Ginekol (Sofiia). 2015;**54**(9): 29-33 [Article in Bulgarian]

[2] International Diabetes Federation. IDF Diabetes Atlas. 9th ed. Brussels, Belgium: International Diabetes Federation; 2019

[3] Hod M, Kapur A, Sacks DA, Hadar E, Agarwal M, Di Renzo GC, et al. The International Federation of Gynecology and Obstetrics (FIGO) initiative on gestational diabetes mellitus: A pragmatic guide for diagnosis, management, and care. International Journal of Gynecology & Obstetrics. 2015;**131**:S173-S211

[4] Dalfrà MG, Nicolucci A, Bisson T, Bonsembiante B, Lapolla A. Quality of life in pregnancy and post-partum: a study in diabetic patients. Quality of Life Research. 2012;**21**(2):291-298

[5] Lapolla A, Di Cianni G, Di Benedetto A, et al. Quality of life, wishes, and needs in women with gestational diabetes: Italian DAWN pregnancy study. International Journal of Endocrinology. 2012;**2012**:6

[6] Kim C, Newton KM, Knopp RH. Gestational diabetes and the incidence of type 2 diabetes. Diabetes Care. 2002;**25**(10):1862-1868

[7] Karagiannis T, Bekiari E, Manolopoulos K, Paletas K, Tsapas A. Gestational diabetes mellitus: Why screen and how to diagnose. Hippokratia. 2011;**2**:187

[8] Goldschmidt VJ, Colletta B. The challenges of providing diabetes education in resource-limited settings to women with diabetes in pregnancy: Perspectives of an educator. Diabetes Spectrum: A Publication of the American Diabetes Association. 2016;**29**(2):101-104

[9] Todorova K. Diabetes and pregnancy. 1st ed. Sofia: Artik; 2010 [In Bulgarian]

[10] Diabetes Legends: Dr. Elliot Proctor Joslin – A Pioneer of Diabetes Treatment. Available from: https://www.diabetes.co.uk/blog/2015/06/diabetes-legends-dr-elliot-proctor-joslin/ [Accessed: 20 August 2021]

[11] Dunn PM. Dr Priscilla White (1900-1989) of Boston and pregnancy diabetes. Archives of Disease in Childhood. Fetal and Neonatal Edition. 2004;**89**(3):F276-F278

[12] Holt T, Kumar S. Helping people live with diabetes. In: ABC of Diabetes. 7th ed. Chichester, West Sussex: Wiley-Blackwell; 2015. pp. 11-14

[13] Okun S, Schoenbaum SC, Andrews D, et al. 2014. Patients and health care teams forging effective partnerships. NAM Perspectives. Discussion Paper, National Academy of Medicine. Available from: https://nam.edu/perspectives-2014-patients-and-health-care-teams-forging-effective-partnerships/. [Accessed: 01 September 2021]

[14] Rhee M, Cook C, El-Kobbi I, Lyles R, et al. Barriers to diabetes education in urban patients. Perceptions, patterns, and associated factors. The Diabetes Educator. 2005;**31**(3):410-417

[15] IDF School of Diabetes. Available from: https://www.idfdiabeteschool.org [Accessed: 20 August 2021]

[16] Tankova T. Diabetes Mellitus. 1st ed. Sofia: Paradigma; 2013 [In Bulgarian]

[17] Golay A, Lagger G, Chambauleyron M, et al. Therapeutic

education of diabetic patients. Diabetes/Metabolism Research and Reviews. 2008;**24**(3):192-196

[18] Cochran J, Conn VS. Meta-analysis of quality of life outcomes following diabetes self-management training. The Diabetes Educator. 2008;**34**(5):815-823

[19] Duncan I, Ahmed T, Li Q, Stetson B, Ruggiero L, Burton K, et al. Assessing the value of the diabetes educator. The Diabetes Educator. 2011;**37**(5):638-657

[20] Robbins JM, Thatcher GE, Webb DA, Valdmanis VG. Nutritionist visits, diabetes classes, and hospitalization rates and charges. Diabetes Care. 2008;**31**(4):655-660

[21] Wizowski L, Harper T, Hutchings T. Writing Health Information for Patients and Families: A Guide to Creating Patient Education Materials that are Easy to Read, Understand and Use. 4th ed. Hamilton, ON, Canada: Hamilton Health Sciences; 2014

[22] Hoffmann T, Warrall L. Designing effective written health education materials: Considerations for health professionals. Disability and Rehabilitation. 2004;**26**(9):1166-1173

[23] Lebanova H, Getov I. Adapted methodology for development and evaluation of patients' educational materials for pharmacovigilance. Academia. 2013;**3**:35-37

[24] Oliveira SC, Lopes MV, Fernandes AF. Development and validation of an educational booklet for healthy eating during pregnancy. Revista Latino-Americana de Enfermagem. 2014;**22**(4):611-620

[25] IDF, E-library, Guidelines. Available from: https://www.idf.org/e-library/guidelines/97-having-a-baby-now-is-the-time-to-learn-more-about-gestational-diabetes.html [Accessed: 01 September 2021]

[26] Chaparro M. Pregnancy & Diabetes: A Complete Guide for Women with Gestational, Type 2, and Type 1 Diabetes. 1st ed. Alexandria (VA): American Diabetes Association; 2020

[27] CDC. Diabetes and Pregnancy – Gestational Diabetes. Available from: https://www.cdc.gov/pregnancy/documents/Diabetes_and_Pregnancy508.pdf [Accessed: 01 September 2021]

[28] NDSS. Gestational Diabetes: Caring for Yourself and Your Baby. Available from: https://www.ndss.com.au/wp-content/uploads/resources/booklet-gestational-diabetes-caring-for-yourself-and-baby.pdf [Accessed: 01 September 2021]

[29] Staynova R. Gestational Diabetes Mellitus – Manual for Healthy Pregnancy. 1st ed. Sofia: TEA Design Ltd.; 2017 [In Bulgarian]

[30] Staynova RA, Gueorguiev SR, Petkova-Gueorguieva ES, Vasileva EV, Stoimenova AH, Yanatchkova VE, et al. Written health education materials for women with gestational diabetes mellitus—Evaluation of usefulness and patients' satisfaction. Folia Medica. 2019;**61**:117

[31] Craig J, Petterson V. Introduction to the practice of telemedicine. Journal of Telemedicine and Telecare. 2005;**11**(1):3-9

[32] Galiero R, Pafundi PC, Nevola R, Rinaldi L, Acierno C, Caturano A, et al. The importance of telemedicine during COVID-19 pandemic: A focus on diabetic retinopathy. Journal of Diabetes Research. 2020;**2020**:1-8

[33] Reicher S, Sela T, Toren O. Using telemedicine during the COVID-19 pandemic: Attitudes of adult health care consumers in Israel. Frontiers in Public Health. 2021;**9**:653553

[34] Aberer F, Hochfellner DA, Mader JK. Application of telemedicine in diabetes care: The time is now. Diabetes Therapy. 2021;**12**(3):629-639

[35] Xie W, Dai P, Qin Y, Wu M, Yang B, Yu X. Effectiveness of telemedicine for pregnant women with gestational diabetes mellitus: An updated meta-analysis of 32 randomized controlled trials with trial sequential analysis. BMC Pregnancy and Childbirth. 2020; **20**(1):1-4

[36] Sayakhot P, Carolan-Olah M, Steele C. Use of a web-based educational intervention to improve knowledge of healthy diet and lifestyle in women with gestational diabetes mellitus compared to standard clinic-based education. BMC Pregnancy and Childbirth. 2016;**16**(1):1-2

[37] Carolan-Olah M, Steele C, Krenzin G. Development and initial testing of a GDM information website for multi-ethnic women with GDM. BMC Pregnancy and Childbirth. 2015;**15**(1):1-9

[38] Carolan-Olah M, Sayakhot P. A randomized controlled trial of a web-based education intervention for women with gestational diabetes mellitus. Midwifery. 2019;**68**:39-47

[39] Miremberg H, Ben-Ari T, Betzer T, et al. The impact of a daily smartphone-based feedback system among women with gestational diabetes on compliance, glycemic control, satisfaction, and pregnancy outcome: A randomized controlled trial. American Journal of Obstetrics and Gynecology. 2018; **218**:453.e1-453.e7

[40] Immanuel J, Simmons D. Apps and the woman with gestational diabetes mellitus. Diabetes Care. 2021;**44**(2): 313-315

[41] Zahmatkeshan M, Zakerabasali S, Farjam M, Gholampour Y, Seraji M, Yazdani A. The use of mobile health interventions for gestational diabetes mellitus: A descriptive literature review. Journal of Medicine and Life. 2021;**14**(2):131

[42] Tassone C, Keshavjee K, Paglialonga A, Moreira N, Pinto J, Quintana Y. Evaluation of mobile apps for treatment of patients at risk of developing gestational diabetes. Health Informatics Journal. 2020;**26**(3): 1983-1994

[43] Guo H, Zhang Y, Li P, Zhou P, Chen LM, Li SY. Evaluating the effects of mobile health intervention on weight management, glycemic control and pregnancy outcomes in patients with gestational diabetes mellitus. Journal of Endocrinological Investigation. 2019;**42**(6):709-714

[44] Mackillop L, Hirst JE, Bartlett KJ, Birks JS, Clifton L, Farmer AJ, et al. Comparing the efficacy of a mobile phone-based blood glucose management system with standard clinic care in women with gestational diabetes: Randomized controlled trial. JMIR mHealth and uHealth. 2018;**6**(3): e9512

[45] Al-Ofi EA, Mosli HH, Ghamri KA, Ghazali SM. Management of postprandial hyperglycaemia and weight gain in women with gestational diabetes mellitus using a novel telemonitoring system. Journal of International Medical Research. 2019;**47**(2):754-764

[46] Yew TW, Chi C, Chan SY, van Dam RM, Whitton C, Lim CS, et al. A randomized controlled trial to evaluate the effects of a smartphone application-based lifestyle coaching program on gestational weight gain, glycemic control, and maternal and neonatal outcomes in women with gestational diabetes mellitus: The SMART-GDM study. Diabetes Care. 2021;**44**(2): 456-463

Chapter 5

Using Resistance Training in Women with Gestational Diabetes Mellitus to Improve Glucose Regulation

Brittany R. Allman, Samantha McDonald, Linda May, Amber W. Kinsey and Elisabet Børsheim

Abstract

Gestational diabetes mellitus (GDM) poses a significant threat to the short- and long-term health of the mother and baby. Pharmacological treatments for GDM do not fully correct the underlying problem of the disease; however, non-pharmacological treatments such as exercise are increasingly recognized as foundational to glycemic management in other populations with disordered glucose regulation, such as non-gravid women with type II diabetes mellitus (T2DM). Much of the research regarding the impact of exercise on glycemic control in T2DM leverages aerobic training as the primary modality; yet research has demonstrated the effectiveness of resistance training on improving glycemic control in T2DM. This chapter will review the rationale for resistance training in the management of GDM using evidence from individuals with T2DM; then the chapter will review available studies on the effectiveness of resistance training on glucose control in women with GDM.

Keywords: physical activity, pregnancy, aerobic training, resistance training, strength training, insulin, glucose, insulin resistance, insulin sensitivity

1. Introduction

Gestational diabetes mellitus (GDM) is glucose intolerance diagnosed during pregnancy [1] and occurs in approximately 10% of all pregnancies [2]. The prevalence of GMD is increasing in the United States [3, 4] and once diagnosed, the odds of GDM in subsequent pregnancies [5, 6] and postpartum type II diabetes mellitus (T2DM) [7, 8] are significantly increased. GDM poses significant health threats to mothers and their offspring, including, but not limited to, placental dysfunction, preterm birth, neural tube defects, macrosomia [9, 10], and increased cardiometabolic disease risk (e.g., obesity, insulin resistance) later in life [11–14]. Consequently, the threat of declining, preventable health outcomes of future generations is imminent, prompting the need for cost-effective therapeutic strategies for the treatment of GDM. Exercise is an effective lifestyle intervention for GDM; however, the precise design of such interventions first requires an understanding of the metabolic changes that occur during pregnancy and the development of GDM.

2. Metabolic changes in pregnancy and the development of GDM

From conception to birth, the female human body undergoes several structural and physiological changes to optimize fetal growth and development; these changes related to normal gestation have been extensively reviewed by others [15]. In uncomplicated pregnancies, maternal metabolism adjusts to the nutrient and energy needs of the growing fetus. In the first half of pregnancy, the fetal nutrient and energy demand is rather low. Thus, maternal metabolism is in an anabolic state favoring nutrient storage, demonstrated by enhanced appetite and tissue-specific insulin sensitivity, specifically of adipose tissue (i.e., fat tissue), and consequently increases in stored triglycerides [15].

Conversely, from the mid-2nd trimester until birth, there is a rapid acceleration in fetal nutrient and energy demands paralleling the augmented growth and development, requiring another shift in maternal metabolism [15]. In this phase, maternal metabolism shifts from an anabolic state to a catabolic state characterized by marked increases in maternal insulin resistance and the shunting of maternal glucose to the fetus, which is the most critical energy substrate for optimal fetal growth and development [15]. Maternal insulin resistance primarily occurs within the skeletal muscle, resulting in progressive and substantial reductions (~55–75%) in maternal glucose uptake relative to pre-pregnancy [15]. Subsequently, meeting the energy demands of the mother requires a dramatic increase in lipolysis, specifically of the triglyceride stores deposited in early pregnancy [16, 17]. Paralleling the increase in maternal insulin resistance, maternal serum lipid concentrations increase by 200–300% compared to pre-pregnancy [16, 17]. The natural increases in maternal insulin resistance must occur or its absence leads to severe fetal growth restriction and permanent, lifelong adverse health outcomes.

The onset of maternal insulin resistance prompts the maternal pancreas to upregulate insulin production and secretion, promoting adequate, yet still reduced, maternal glucose uptake. This response maintains optimal fetal glucose supply, protecting it from an oversupply. However, a failed or insufficient pancreatic response and increased maternal glucose concentrations may lead to a persistent state of maternal hyperglycemia, yielding a continuous oversupply of glucose to the fetus. Consequently, the maternal pancreas either (1) continues to respond to the hyperglycemia via further increases in insulin production and secretion resulting in maternal hyperinsulinemia potentially worsening the progressing maternal insulin resistance and ensuing hyperglycemia via reduced insulin receptor sensitivity or (2) fails to produce and secrete a sufficient amount of maternal insulin, yielding worsened hyperglycemia, without hyperinsulinemia. These alterations in maternal metabolic responses can lead to the development and diagnosis of GDM.

Given the grave maternal and fetal health consequences of glucose intolerance and GDM, all pregnant women are screened for glucose intolerance or GDM in the mid-to-late 2nd trimester via glucose challenge tests by consuming a beverage containing a 50-g load of glucose. Following intake, maternal blood is drawn via venipuncture and serum glucose levels measured. If maternal fasting glucose levels exceed 95 mg dL^{-1}, or if glucose levels at 1-h post-dose exceed 180 mg dL^{-1}, the pregnant women 'fails' and subsequently undergoes a 3-h glucose oral glucose tolerance test (OGTT) to confirm a GDM diagnosis. To confirm a GDM diagnosis, maternal glucose levels must exceed two of the following three glucose thresholds: 180 mg dL^{-1} at 1 h, 155 mg dL^{-1} at 2 h, or 140 mg dL^{-1} at 3 h post OGTT [18]. A confirmed GDM diagnosis requires immediate treatment intervention.

3. Current treatment interventions for GDM

The first line of treatment for GDM includes medical nutrition therapy (e.g., complex carbohydrate-rich diabetic diet), capillary blood glucose monitoring, and recommendations of at least 150 min of aerobic exercise per week [18]. If clinicians render the behavioral strategies ineffective, pharmacological therapy (insulin, metformin, or glyburide) is prescribed [18]. Pharmacological therapy effectively manages maternal hyperglycemia via stimulation of peripheral glucose uptake by skeletal muscle and fat cells, and by inhibiting hepatic glucose production. While effective, pharmacological therapies fail to address the underlying mechanisms that cause insulin resistance in GDM, including a reduction in peripheral and hepatic insulin sensitivity, pancreatic β-cell failure or damage, and dysfunctional insulin action at the post-receptor level in skeletal muscle [19]. Furthermore, pharmacological therapy is associated with adverse health outcomes such as small-for-gestational-age offspring [20] and maternal vascular damage [21], and comes with a significant medical financial burden.

In contrast, exercise has been shown to improve peripheral (e.g., muscle) glucose tolerance through both insulin-dependent and insulin-independent mechanisms [22], and pancreatic β-cell function [23, 24] in T2DM populations. With this general understanding of the benefits of exercise for glucose management, several professional organizations such as the American College of Obstetrics and Gynecology [25], the American College of Sports Medicine [26], the American Diabetes Association [27] advocate for the use of prenatal exercise as an adjunctive therapy to improve glycemia in GDM.

4. Exercise and GDM

4.1 Exercise and aerobic exercise: definitions

Exercise training is defined as a structured, goal-oriented, progressive behavioral regimen, whereby individuals repeatedly perform bodily movements aimed to improve health, locomotion, ease of daily physical activities, sports performance etc. Two common types of exercise training are aerobic training and resistance training. Aerobic training involves performing exercises that rhythmically and continuously move large muscle groups for sustained periods of time such as walking, cycling, rowing, swimming, running etc. Aerobic training typically focuses on improving an individual's cardiorespiratory fitness.

4.2 Resistance training: definition

Resistance training is a form of exercise characterized by repetitive voluntary skeletal muscle contractions working against an external resistance (e.g., gravity during body weight exercises, free weights) and is designed to improve muscular fitness [28]. Resistance training programs typically focus on improving muscular strength. One form of resistance training, called strength training, typically involves higher loads (e.g., heavier weight), lower repetitions, more recovery time between sets, and isolates specific muscle groups (e.g., legs, back). For example, a person might perform a barbell squat at 75% of their maximal effort for three sets of 8 repetitions, with 2 min of rest between sets. Circuit training is a form of body conditioning involving full-body exercises performed in a series with minimal rest between each exercise. Although it is predominately a form a resistance training, circuit training often includes a combination of resistance training and moderate-to-high intensity aerobic training. Circuit resistance training typically involves lighter loads or body weight, a higher number of repetitions (e.g., 10–15), and little to no rest periods. One example of CRT might be performing the following eight exercises for 10 repetitions each, as many times as possible in a given amount of time (e.g., 10 min), and taking breaks as needed: chest press, low row, squat, lunge, shoulder press, latissimus dorsi pull-down, biceps curl, and triceps extension.

4.3 Effectiveness of aerobic training in women with GDM

Growing evidence demonstrates that participating in aerobic training during pregnancy elicits profound positive effects on maternal glucose tolerance. Previous studies showed that exercising during the first 20 weeks of pregnancy significantly reduces (up to 50%) a pregnant woman's risk of developing GDM [29]. Moreover, studies have shown that prenatal aerobic exercise effectively manages maternal glucose levels and may replace pharmacological therapies in pregnant women diagnosed with GDM [29–31]. For these reasons, several worldwide private and governmental agencies endorse pregnant women engaging in prenatal aerobic exercise for the prevention and management of GDM [24–26], along with a plethora of other health-related benefits. Aerobic training is a promising modality to optimize maternal and offspring outcomes considering this type of exercise encompasses a wide range of activities (e.g., walking, cycling, and swimming).

4.4 Prevalence of resistance training and recommendations

Currently, it is unknown what percentage of pregnant women with GDM participate in resistance training. However, despite being the third most commonly reported activity during pregnancy, resistance training is performed in only 10% of pregnant women overall [32]. These statistics are slightly outdated, however, there have been no other more recent reports over the past several years. Nevertheless, resistance training has gained significant popularity among non-gravid women [33, 34], indicating that women, in general, are becoming more interested in the benefits gleaned from resistance training. However, the lack of resistance training participation while pregnant is likely driven by many factors. Misconceptions about resistance training during pregnancy, in particular, may be a major contributor. For example, anecdotally, common misconceptions include e.g., resistance training being dangerous for the mother and baby, core training causing separation of the abdominal muscles (diastasis recti), an increase in pregnancy pains when resistance training, you cannot perform resistance training during pregnancy if you have never resistance trained before, you cannot lay on your back during exercise after 16 weeks gestation, and others. Although many of these misconceptions are likely rooted in cultural ideologies, the lack of rigorous research regarding the impact of resistance training during pregnancy, especially GDM, is likely the reason that American governing bodies have just recently (year 2020) added resistance training guidelines for all pregnant women [25, 35], and have not yet added resistance training as part of the first line of glucose management upon GDM diagnoses [18, 27]. As a result, the breadth of exercise recommendations at the practice level (e.g., OB/GYNs) is limited. Thus, more research on resistance training in GDM populations is needed to inform the public and in turn impact the participation of pregnant women in resistance training.

4.5 Effectiveness of resistance training in T2DM

Despite a dearth of resistance training research in pregnant women, there is evidence demonstrating the effectiveness of resistance training in individuals with

T2DM, who have similar peripheral impairments in insulin resistance as GDM. For instance, both resistance training and aerobic training individually elicit similar improvements in glycemic control in T2DM in non-gravid adults [36–39], indicating that resistance training may be a novel approach to achieving the same outcome in GDM women. A meta-analysis of studies in GDM [38] determined that as long as the exercise training (either aerobic training or resistance training) is performed at a sufficient frequency (3–4 times per week), intensity (moderate to vigorous), and duration (20–30 min), similar glycemic outcomes will occur in response to aerobic training vs. resistance training. These findings confirm evidence demonstrating mechanical contraction of muscle, in general, is a potent physiological stimulator of skeletal muscle glucose uptake [40], and suggest that the type of exercise (e.g., resistance training or aerobic training) may not be as important given that bodily movement produces muscle contractions. However, glucose uptake into muscle is contraction-intensity dependent in both fast- and slow-twitch skeletal muscle fibers [40]. Thus, although any type of physical activity will increase glucose uptake due to its respective contractile nature, the magnitude of blood glucose uptake depends on the intensity with which the activity is performed.

Although aerobic exercises is often prescribed for glucose management in T2DM, sustaining continuous activity for 30–60 min at a time may be difficult for these individuals for a number of reasons (e.g., reduced aerobic capacity and exercise tolerance, orthopedic issues, excess weight [41, 42]). These barriers to aerobic exercise may encourage exercise participation at lower than recommended intensities or lead to exercise dropout. In general some exercise is better than none, however, there is a positive relationship between the intensity at which aerobic exercise is performed and glycemic control in T2DM [43]. Aerobic exercise may need to be performed at a higher intensity than is feasible for many adults with T2DM to sustain. Fortunately, resistance training may address aforementioned barriers associated with aerobic exercise as it can be performed with lower aerobic effort, intensity can be modified in a variety of ways (e.g., load, tempo, exercise progressions and regressions), and the extent to which activities are weight bearing can be adjusted (e.g., free weights vs. machines). Because these aspects are relevant to T2DM and pregnant women, resistance training may be an effective exercise option for GDM populations.

On a practical level, it may not be prudent to simply recommend an increase in physical activity (e.g., walk more throughout the day) in patients with glucose regulatory disorders, such as GDM. Nevertheless, if the exercise dose (frequency, intensity, and duration) is at or above recommended levels, the type of exercise may not be as important for glucose regulation in GDM. These findings are encouraging for both practitioners and pregnant women since it moves the focus of an exercise program to the preferences of the pregnant woman, allowing the program to be individually tailored. The ability to adjust exercise prescription to the needs and preferences of the individual will ultimately help increase adherence to an exercise program and lifestyle modification.

5. Mechanisms of the improvement in insulin sensitivity with resistance training in T2DM

The mechanisms by which resistance training may improve glycemia in GDM has not yet been elucidated in the literature. Therefore, this section will review the mechanisms of resistance training-induced improvements in glycemia in T2DM. The improvements in glycemia with resistance training can occur independent of the addition of aerobic training into a resistance training program [44], and without changes in maximal oxygen uptake [45]. In other words, improved insulin sensitivity with resistance training can occur without improved aerobic capacity suggesting that resistance training alone may be a sufficient stimulus to improve glycemia independent of traditional aerobic exercise training recommendations for the management of glycemia. In fact, studies have reported that the impact of resistance training on insulin sensitivity and glucose control is greater than aerobic training [46, 47], or at a minimum, elicits the same glycemic effect [48], when matched for training units or time. Therefore, it may be that the higher intensity contractile nature of resistance training compared to aerobic training results in greater glucose uptake during exercise, and this physiological stimulus may supersede the benefit of improved aerobic capacity on glycemia.

There are a variety of reported mechanisms by which resistance training improves glucose regulation in T2DM. First, resistance training increases muscular glucose disposal and insulin sensitivity [49, 50], which can occur acutely after a singular resistance training session [51]. However, resistance training should be maintained as a part of a regular exercise routine because the effect of resistance training on glycemic control and insulin sensitivity is not sustained when resistance training is discontinued [52]. Second, although it may be assumed that hypertrophy is one of the mechanisms by which glucose control is achieved with chronic resistance training in T2DM, an increase in muscle mass, *per se*, may not be the direct catalyst of change [53]. Instead, an array of intrinsic metabolic changes within the muscle may be the driver of improvements in glucose control in T2DM. For instance, resistance training increases insulin receptor concentration [54] and enhances the activation of the insulin signaling cascade [55, 56]. Upon activation of insulin receptors by insulin, several intracellular cascades are stimulated, including glucose transporter type 4 (GLUT4) translocation that ultimately increases glucose uptake into the cell. GLUT4 permits facilitated diffusion of glucose into skeletal muscles, and therefore, a larger concentration of GLUT4 and faster movement of GLUT4 to the cell surface with resistance training will enhance glucose flux into the cell, and therefore better regulate blood glucose levels. Resistance training also directly increases the content and rate of GLUT4 translocation within the muscle cell [57]. Importantly, these changes occur independent of significant increases in muscle mass [58], and even after only one resistance training session or single set of exercises [51], suggesting that repeated mechanical muscular contractions, rather than muscle growth, may be the most important for glucose control in T2DM. These findings, however, should not discount the importance of muscle mass, because it is known that low relative muscle mass is related to an increased risk of developing T2DM [59]. However, these findings may be particularly important for pregnant women, considering that (1) there is a stigma around resistance training and becoming "bulky" in female populations, and (2) resistance training programs may not have to be built on high intensity regimens (i.e., it does not have to be straining) characteristic of muscle hypertrophy programs to achieve glycemic benefits. Considering there is a substantial body of evidence to suggest that resistance training is beneficial for glycemic control in T2DM, and the peripheral insulin resistance effects of T2DM and GDM are similar, it may be assumed that many of the mechanisms of change as a result of resistance training in GDM would be similar to T2DM. However, mechanistic data in women with GDM is not available in the current literature. Therefore, the next section will discuss available research on the effect of resistance training on several clinical outcomes related to glucose control. Future research describing the mechanisms by which these changes occur is needed.

6. The effect of resistance training on glucose regulation in GDM

6.1 Risk of GDM

It is important to determine the impact of resistance training during pregnancy on the risk of developing GDM to evaluate resistance training as preventative therapy, rather than solely for treatment upon diagnosis. However, the only reported study that assessed this relationship found that a moderate intensity resistance training intervention during pregnancy did not reduce the risk of developing GDM in sedentary, normal weight Spanish women after adjusting for maternal age and body weight pre-pregnancy [60]. Therefore, it may be that light-to-moderate intensity resistance training exercises cannot "override" the predisposition that women with higher BMIs (even though the ones in the study were normal weight) have for the risk of GDM. This study was limited because it assessed healthy women with normal BMIs, and not overweight or obese women who are known to have a significantly higher risk of developing GDM [61]. In addition, the resistance training protocol (3×/wk., 25–30 min per session at moderate intensity) included "toning and joint mobilization," which consisted of isolation movements of small muscles or muscle groups using very light loads (3 kg barbells and 1–3 kg elastic resistance bands). The movements included shoulder shrugs and rotations, arm elevations, leg lateral elevations, and pelvic tilts and rocks. Women who are experienced weightlifters would consider this protocol to be more of a mobility and activation routine characteristic of a warm-up, rather than a workout routine that properly stresses the muscle. Depending on an individual's experience with resistance training, the light-to-moderate intensity exercises described in the study may not provide a sufficient mechanical stimulus to evoke changes at the level of the muscle. The women in the study mentioned above were sedentary; therefore, they may have initially gleaned strength benefits from the program, but likely would have quickly plateaued. Even so, this particular study did not assess muscular strength gains as a result of the resistance training intervention. The goal of the study may not have been to use traditional resistance training with the goal of improving strength considering it was designed for toning and mobilization. Overall, more research is needed to determine if a resistance training program providing a sufficient stimulus reduces the risk of GDM in at-risk women, such as women with overweight and obesity or those with a history of GDM.

6.2 Insulin therapy

It may not be viable to use resistance training as a preventative therapy against the diagnosis of GDM in all women because there may be a low likelihood of starting a resistance training exercise routine prior to conception in women with no prior experience in resistance training. Therefore, determining how resistance training can attenuate the pharmacological requirement for the regulation of glucose in women with GDM upon diagnosis is important. Insulin therapy is the first line antihyperglycemic drug therapy recommended for treatment of GDM [62] when initial lifestyle changes (medical nutrition therapy, physical activity) are ineffective. One study demonstrated that fewer women in the resistance training group required insulin therapy compared to the control group [63]; while another study found no differences between resistance training-plus-diet vs. diet alone (standard diabetic diet) groups [64]. However, all women in the resistance training-plus-diet group were prescribed less insulin (diet: 0.48 ± 0.3 units/kg; resistance training-plus-diet: 0.22 ± 0.2 units/kg, $P < 0.05$) and commenced insulin therapy later after diagnosis (diet: 1.1 ± 0.8 weeks;

resistance training-plus-diet: 3.71 ± 3.1 weeks, $P < 0.05$) [64]. Furthermore, overweight women in the resistance training-plus-diet group had a significantly lower incidence of insulin therapy use [64]. Therefore, the effect of diet therapy on insulin use may be complemented by the addition of resistance training overall, and the metabolic effects of resistance training are likely to be greater in women with higher BMIs compared to women with healthy weight BMI. These findings are of no surprise considering it is likely that the diabetic diet consisting of less daily carbohydrates (40% of total energy intake) and the contractile nature of resistance training have a synergistic effect on the maintenance of blood glucose levels. Although both diet and exercise are the first line of treatment for GDM, this study was the only one to combine exercise and nutrition therapy. Therefore, more research that truly reflects the overall treatment strategies for women with GDM is required.

6.3 Fasting glucose and insulin concentrations

Being one of the most widely used clinical measures of glycemia, fasting glucose and insulin concentrations must be examined with a resistance training intervention during GDM. The American Diabetes Association recommends that fasting glucose concentrations during pregnancy should be <95 mg dL^{-1} [27]. After chronic resistance training in women with GDM, fasting glucose concentration tends to decrease more from pre- to post-intervention compared to aerobic training [63, 65–67]. However there are rarely differences between resistance training and aerobic training groups [63, 65–68], indicating that exercise in general (e.g., muscular contraction) may be the most important factor in the regulation of fasting glucose concentrations. Importantly, although the women in each of these studies were diagnosed with GDM, they had well-managed glucose levels represented by fasting glucose concentrations below recommended levels even before the exercise intervention. Thus, perhaps women with GDM with less control over circulating glucose concentrations may be more responsive to exercise training. In regard to fasting insulin concentrations, most work has demonstrated that there is no effect of resistance training [65, 69], however, one study showed a significant difference between resistance training and aerobic training groups whereby fasting insulin levels increased with resistance training and decreased with aerobic training [66]. Nevertheless, fasting insulin levels after the resistance training intervention (10.22 ± 2.76 mIU/mL) were still within normal limits (<20 mIU/L [70]). Therefore, it seems that there are minimal to no effects of resistance training on fasting insulin concentrations in GDM.

6.4 Markers of insulin resistance and β-cell function

A more significant indicator of the potential impact of resistance training on glucose regulation in GDM may be indirect measures of insulin resistance and pancreatic beta cell function. For example, measures such as the homeostatic model assessment (HOMA) of insulin resistance (HOMA-IR) and HOMA-β, respectively, use fasting insulin and glucose concentrations. The only reference values for HOMA-IR during pregnancy are in Mexican women (first trimester: <1.6; second trimester: <2.9, third trimester: <2.6) [71], however, in general, the higher the HOMA-IR values, the more insulin resistant the individual. Changes in HOMA-IR tends to not differ between resistance training and aerobic training protocols in GDM [65, 69]; however, one study found there was a significant difference between resistance training, aerobic training, and control groups, with HOMA-IR decreasing to a greater extent in the aerobic training (−7.1%) compared to resistance training (−3.54%) groups. Nonetheless, HOMA-IR was reduced in both exercise groups and increased in the non-exercise control group (+9.06%), indicating that, much like fasting glucose concentrations, exercise in general (and not exercise type) may be the most important factor regulating indirect measures of insulin resistance in GDM. On the other hand, in the few studies using HOMA-β, an estimate of steady-state beta-cell function, no differences have been found between resistance training, aerobic training, and control groups [65, 66]. Therefore, more research is needed to assess the impact of resistance training on β-cell function.

The impact of resistance training in women with GDM on dynamic measures of glycemia, such as post-meal and post-exercise glucose concentrations, are promising. Chronic resistance training in women with GDM is associated with a greater percentage of weeks spent within a healthy target glucose range throughout the day (e.g. after an overnight fast, and after meals) compared to no exercise [63]. In addition, women with GDM using insulin therapy and exercise also spent more weeks within a healthy target glucose range throughout the day compared to women using insulin therapy that do not exercise [63]. Another study confirmed that after chronic resistance training in women with GDM, there is a greater reduction in postprandial glucose levels compared to aerobic training [68]; these findings indicating that resistance training may improve nutrient handling after a meal to a greater extent than aerobic training. Lastly, there are no differences in the reduction in blood glucose levels from baseline between an acute bout of resistance training vs. aerobic training [67], indicating that resistance training is a safe exercise modality to use in women with GDM, especially as it pertains to post-exercise glucose levels. Therefore, overall, resistance training in women with GDM improves glycemia throughout the day, and specifically after a meal, indicating that it may have therapeutic potential for women with GDM.

7. Conclusions

In conclusion, because of the potent effects of resistance training on glucose control in T2DM, it may be surmised that resistance training would also benefit women with GDM, who share similar impairments in peripheral insulin resistance. However, the studies of resistance training in women with GDM are minimal. Based on the work available, there seems to be initial promise for the use of resistance training in women with GDM to reduce the need for pharmacological insulin and improve glucose control throughout the day and after meals. Future work should assess the impact of a resistance training program on the risk of GDM in women with obesity; additionally, future research should provide more knowledge about potential effects of resistance training on clinical outcomes such as glucose and markers of insulin resistance. As more research becomes available, exercise guidelines can be properly tailored to pregnant women in a way that includes not only AT, but also resistance training.

Acknowledgements

The Arkansas Children's Research Institute and Arkansas Biosciences Institute Postgraduate Grant (B.R.A.).

Conflict of interest

B.R.A. has a podcast about exercise and health-related outcomes ("BENT by Knowledge") and is also the Senior Innovation Scientist for Breakout Lifestyle

Fitness, Little Rock, a gym emphasizing resistance training and health-related outcomes. The other authors report no conflicts of interest or competing interests.

Appendices and nomenclature

BMI	body mass index
GDM	gestational diabetes mellitus
GLUT4	glucose transporter protein type 4
HOMA-β	homeostatic model assessment of beta cell function
HOMA-IR	homeostatic model assessment of insulin resistance
T2DM	Type II diabetes mellitus

Author details

Brittany R. Allman[1,2,3*], Samantha McDonald[4], Linda May[5,6,7], Amber W. Kinsey[8] and Elisabet Børsheim[1,2,3,9]

1 Arkansas Children's Nutrition Center, Little Rock, AR, USA

2 Arkansas Children's Research Institute, Little Rock, AR, USA

3 Department of Pediatrics, University of Arkansas for Medical Sciences, Little Rock, AR, USA

4 School of Kinesiology and Recreation, Illinois State University, Normal, IL, USA

5 Department of Obstetrics and Gynecology, East Carolina University (ECU), Greenville, NC, USA

6 Department of Kinesiology, ECU, Greenville, NC, USA

7 Department of Foundational Sciences and Research, ECU, Greenville, NC, USA

8 Department of Medicine, Division of Preventive Medicine, University of Alabama at Birmingham, Birmingham, AL, USA

9 Departments of Geriatrics, University of Arkansas for Medical Sciences, Little Rock, AR, USA

*Address all correspondence to: ballman@uams.edu

References

[1] Proceedings of the 4th International Workshop-Conference on Gestational Diabetes Mellitus. Chicago, Illinois, USA. 14-16. March 1997. Diabetes Care. 1998;**21 Suppl 2**:B1-B167

[2] DeSisto CL, Kim SY, Sharma AJ. Prevalence estimates of gestational diabetes mellitus in the United States, Pregnancy Risk Assessment Monitoring System (PRAMS), 2007-2010. Preventing Chronic Disease. 2014; **11**:E104. DOI: 10.5888/pcd11.130415

[3] American Diabetes Association. Standards of medical care in diabetes—2015. Diabetes Care. 2015;**38**: S1-S2. DOI: 10.2337/dc15-S001

[4] Practice Bulletin No. 137: Gestational diabetes mellitus. Obstetrics Gynecology. 2013;**122**:406-416. DOI: 10.1097/01.AOG.0000433006.09219.f1

[5] Gaudier FL, Hauth JC, Poist M, Corbett D, Cliver SP. Recurrence of gestational diabetes mellitus. Obstetrics and Gynecology. 1992;**80**:755-758

[6] Moses RG. The recurrence rate of gestational diabetes in subsequent pregnancies. Diabetes Care. 1996;**19**: 1348-1350. DOI: 10.2337/diacare. 19.12.1348

[7] O'Sullivan JB. Diabetes mellitus after GDM. Diabetes. 1991;**40**(Suppl 2): 131-135. DOI: 10.2337/diab.40.2.s131

[8] Henry OA, Beischer NA. Long-term implications of gestational diabetes for the mother. Baillière's Clinical Obstetrics and Gynaecology. 1991;**5**:461-483. DOI: 10.1016/s0950-3552(05)80107-5

[9] Leddy MA, Power ML, Schulkin J. The impact of maternal obesity on maternal and fetal health. Reviews in Obstetrics and Gynecology. 2008; **1**:170-178

[10] Lynch CM, Sexton DJ, Hession M, Morrison JJ. Obesity and mode of delivery in primigravid and multigravid women. American Journal of Perinatology. 2008;**25**:163-167. DOI: 10.1055/s-2008-1061496

[11] Freeman DJ. Effects of maternal obesity on fetal growth and body composition: Implications for programming and future health. Seminars in Fetal and Neonatal Medicine. 2010;**15**:113-118. DOI: 10.1016/j.siny.2009.09.001

[12] Catalano PM, Presley L, Minium J, Hauguel-de MS. Fetuses of obese mothers develop insulin resistance in utero. Diabetes Care. 2009;**32**:1076-1080. DOI: 10.2337/dc08-2077

[13] Whitaker RC. Predicting preschooler obesity at birth: The role of maternal obesity in early pregnancy. Pediatrics. 2004;**114**:e29-e36. DOI: 10.1542/peds.114.1.e29

[14] Schmatz M, Madan J, Marino T, Davis J. Maternal obesity: The interplay between inflammation, mother and fetus. Journal of Perinatology. 2010;**30**: 441-446. DOI: 10.1038/jp.2009.182

[15] Hytten F, Chamberlain G. Clinical Physiology in Obstetrics. Oxford, United Kingdom: Blackwell Scientific Publications; 1980

[16] Knopp RH, Herrera E, Freinkel N. Carbohydrate metabolism in pregnancy. 8. Metabolism of adipose tissue isolated from fed and fasted pregnant rats during late gestation. The Journal of Clinical Investigation. 1970;**49**:1438-1446. DOI: 10.1172/JCI106361

[17] Grimes SB, Wild R. Effect of pregnancy on lipid metabolism and lipoprotein levels [Online]. In: Feingold KR, Anawalt B, Boyce A, Chrousos G, de Herder WW,

Dhatariya K, et al. editors. Endotext. MDText.com, Inc; 2021. Available from: http://www.ncbi.nlm.nih.gov/books/NBK498654/

[18] Practice Bulletin No ACOG. 190: Gestational diabetes mellitus. Obstetrics and Gynecology. 2018;**131**:e49-e64. DOI: 10.1097/AOG.0000000000002501

[19] Coustan DR. Pharmacological management of gestational diabetes: An overview. Diabetes Care. 2007;**30**: S206-S208. DOI: 10.2337/dc07-s217

[20] Tarry-Adkins JL, Aiken CE, Ozanne SE. Neonatal, infant, and childhood growth following metformin versus insulin treatment for gestational diabetes: A systematic review and meta-analysis. PLoS Medicine. 2019;**16**: e1002848. DOI: 10.1371/journal.pmed.1002848

[21] Meigs JB, Mittleman MA, Nathan DM, Tofler GH, Singer DE, Murphy-Sheehy PM, et al. Hyperinsulinemia, hyperglycemia, and impaired hemostasis: The Framingham Offspring Study. JAMA. 2000;**283**:221-228. DOI: 10.1001/jama.283.2.221

[22] Romeres D, Schiavon M, Basu A, Cobelli C, Basu R, Dalla MC. Exercise effect on insulin-dependent and insulin-independent glucose utilization in healthy individuals and individuals with type 1 diabetes: A modeling study. The American Journal of Physiology—Endocrinology and Metabolism. 2021;**321**:E122-E129. DOI: 10.1152/ajpendo.00084.2021

[23] Dela F, von Linstow ME, Mikines KJ, Galbo H. Physical training may enhance β-cell function in type 2 diabetes. The American Journal of Physiology—Endocrinology and Metabolism. 2004;**287**:E1024-E1031. DOI: 10.1152/ajpendo.00056.2004

[24] Heiskanen MA, Motiani KK, Mari A, Saunavaara V, Eskelinen J-J, Virtanen KA, et al. Exercise training decreases pancreatic fat content and improves beta cell function regardless of baseline glucose tolerance: A randomised controlled trial. Diabetologia. 2018;**61**:1817-1828. DOI: 10.1007/s00125-018-4627-x

[25] Physical Activity and Exercise During Pregnancy and the Postpartum Period [Online]. [date unknown]. Available from: https://www.acog.org/en/clinical/clinical-guidance/committee-opinion/articles/2020/04/physical-activity-and-exercise-during-pregnancy-and-the-postpartum-period [Accessed: 22 June 2021]

[26] Pate R, Pratt M, Blair S, Macera C, Bouchard C, Buchner D, et al. A recommendation from The Centers for Disease Control and Prevention and the American College of Sports Medicine. JAMA. 1995;**273**:402-407. DOI: 10.1001/jama.273.5.402

[27] Management of diabetes in pregnancy: Standards of medical care in diabetes—2019, American Diabetes Association. Diabetes Care. 2019;**42**: S165-S172. DOI: 10.2337/dc19-S014

[28] Fleck S, Kraemer W. Designing Resistance Training Programs. 3rd ed. Champaign, IL: Human Kinetics; 2003

[29] Oteng-Ntim E, Varma R, Croker H, Poston L, Doyle P. Lifestyle interventions for overweight and obese pregnant women to improve pregnancy outcome: Systematic review and meta-analysis. BMC Medicine. 2012;**10**:47. DOI: 10.1186/1741-7015-10-47

[30] Davenport MH, Mottola MF, McManus R, Gratton R. A walking intervention improves capillary glucose control in women with gestational diabetes mellitus: A pilot study. Applied Physiology, Nutrition, and Metabolism. 2008;**33**:511-517. DOI: 10.1139/H08-018

[31] Dipla K, Zafeiridis A, Mintziori G, Boutou AK, Goulis DG, Hackney AC. Exercise as a therapeutic intervention in gestational diabetes mellitus. Endocrine. 2021;**2**:65-78. DOI: 10.3390/endocrines 2020007

[32] White E, Pivarnik J, Pfeiffer K. Resistance training during pregnancy and perinatal outcomes. Journal of Physical Activity and Health. 2014;**11**:1141-1148. DOI: 10.1123/jpah.2012-0350

[33] Hurley BF, Hanson ED, Sheaff AK. Strength training as a countermeasure to aging muscle and chronic disease. Sports Medicine. 2011;**41**:289-306. DOI: 10.2165/11585920-000000000-00000

[34] Trends in Strength Training—United States, 1998-2004 [Online]. [date unknown]. Available from: https://www.cdc.gov/mmwr/preview/mmwrhtml/mm5528a1.htm [Accessed: 13 September 2021]

[35] Bauer P. ACSM Information on Pregnancy Physical Activity [Online]. American College of Sports Medicine; 2020. Available from: https://www.acsm.org/docs/default-source/files-for-resource-library/pregnancy-physical-activity.pdf?sfvrsn=12a73853_4

[36] Niemann MJ, Tucker LA, Bailey BW, Davidson LE. Strength training and insulin resistance: The mediating role of body composition. Journal of Diabetes Research. 2020;**2020**:e7694825. DOI: 10.1155/2020/7694825

[37] Dunstan DW, Puddey IB, Beilin LJ, Burke V, Morton AR, Stanton KG. Effects of a short-term circuit weight training program on glycaemic control in NIDDM. Diabetes Research and Clinical Practice. 1998;**40**:53-61. DOI: 10.1016/s0168-8227(98)00027-8

[38] Harrison AL, Shields N, Taylor NF, Frawley HC. Exercise improves glycaemic control in women diagnosed with gestational diabetes mellitus: A systematic review. Journal of Physiotherapy. 2016;**62**:188-196. DOI: 10.1016/j.jphys.2016.08.003

[39] Wang C, Guelfi KJ, Yang H-X. Exercise and its role in gestational diabetes mellitus. Chronic Diseases and Translational Medicine. 2016;**2**:208-214. DOI: 10.1016/j.cdtm.2016.11.006

[40] Jensen TE, Sylow L, Rose AJ, Madsen AB, Angin Y, Maarbjerg SJ, et al. Contraction-stimulated glucose transport in muscle is controlled by AMPK and mechanical stress but not sarcoplasmatic reticulum Ca2+ release. Molecular Metabalism. 2014;**3**:742-753. DOI: 10.1016/j.molmet.2014.07.005

[41] Nesti L, Pugliese NR, Sciuto P, Natali A. Type 2 diabetes and reduced exercise tolerance: A review of the literature through an integrated physiology approach. Cardiovascular Diabetology. 2020;**19**:134. DOI: 10.1186/s12933-020-01109-1

[42] Gehling DJ, Lecka-Czernik B, Ebraheim NA. Orthopedic complications in diabetes. Bone. 2016;**82**:79-92. DOI: 10.1016/j.bone.2015.07.029

[43] Liubaoerjijin Y, Terada T, Fletcher K, Boulé NG. Effect of aerobic exercise intensity on glycemic control in type 2 diabetes: A meta-analysis of head-to-head randomized trials. Acta Diabetologica. 2016;**53**:769-781. DOI: 10.1007/s00592-016-0870-0

[44] Grøntved A, Rimm EB, Willett WC, Andersen LB, Hu FB. A prospective study of weight training and risk of type 2 diabetes in men. Archives of Internal Medicine. 2012;**172**:1306-1312. DOI: 10.1001/archinternmed.2012.3138

[45] Ishii T, Yamakita T, Sato T, Tanaka S, Fujii S. Resistance training improves insulin sensitivity in NIDDM subjects without altering maximal oxygen

uptake. Diabetes Care. 1998;**21**:1353-1355. DOI: 10.2337/diacare.21.8.1353

[46] Cauza E, Hanusch-Enserer U, Strasser B, Ludvik B, Metz-Schimmerl S, Pacini G, et al. The relative benefits of endurance and strength training on the metabolic factors and muscle function of people with type 2 diabetes mellitus. Archives of Physical Medicine and Rehabilitation. 2005;**86**:1527-1533. DOI: 10.1016/j.apmr.2005.01.007

[47] Bacchi E, Negri C, Targher G, Faccioli N, Lanza M, Zoppini G, et al. Both resistance training and aerobic training reduce hepatic fat content in type 2 diabetic subjects with nonalcoholic fatty liver disease (the RAED2 Randomized Trial). Hepatology. 2013;**58**:1287-1295. DOI: 10.1002/hep.26393

[48] Bacchi E, Negri C, Zanolin ME, Milanese C, Faccioli N, Trombetta M, et al. Metabolic effects of aerobic training and resistance training in type 2 diabetic subjects: A randomized controlled trial (the RAED2 study). Diabetes Care. 2012;**35**:676-682. DOI: 10.2337/dc11-1655

[49] Umpierre D, Pa R, Ck K, Cb L, At Z, Mj A, et al. Physical activity advice only or structured exercise training and association with HbA1c levels in type 2 diabetes: A systematic review and meta-analysis. JAMA. 2011;**305**. DOI: 10.1001/jama.2011.576

[50] Strasser B, Siebert U, Schobersberger W. Resistance training in the treatment of the metabolic syndrome: A systematic review and meta-analysis of the effect of resistance training on metabolic clustering in patients with abnormal glucose metabolism. Sports Medicine. 2010;**40**:397-415.DOI:10.2165/11531380-000000000-00000

[51] Black LE, Swan PD, Alvar BA. Effects of intensity and volume on insulin sensitivity during acute bouts of resistance training. Journal of Strength and Conditioning Research. 2010;**24**:1109-1116. DOI: 10.1519/JSC.0b013e3181cbab6d

[52] Andersen JL, Schjerling P, Andersen LL, Dela F. Resistance training and insulin action in humans: Effects of de-training. The Journal of Physiology. 2003;**551**:1049-1058. DOI: 10.1113/jphysiol.2003.043554

[53] Cauza E, Strehblow C, Metz-Schimmerl S, Strasser B, Hanusch-Enserer U, Kostner K, et al. Effects of progressive strength training on muscle mass in type 2 diabetes mellitus patients determined by computed tomography. Wiener Medizinische Wochenschrift (1946). 2009;**159**:141-147. DOI: 10.1007/s10354-009-0641-4

[54] Strasser B, Pesta D. Resistance training for diabetes prevention and therapy: Experimental findings and molecular mechanisms. BioMed Research International. 2013; **2013**:805217. DOI: 10.1155/2013/805217

[55] Castaneda C, Layne JE, Munoz-Orians L, Gordon PL, Walsmith J, Foldvari M, et al. A randomized controlled trial of resistance exercise training to improve glycemic control in older adults with type 2 diabetes. Diabetes Care. 2002;**25**:2335-2341. DOI: 10.2337/diacare.25.12.2335

[56] Yaspelkis BB. Resistance training improves insulin signaling and action in skeletal muscle. Exercise and Sport Sciences Reviews. 2006;**34**:42-46. DOI: 10.1097/00003677-200601000-00009

[57] Holten MK, Zacho M, Gaster M, Juel C, Wojtaszewski JFP, Dela F. Strength training increases insulin-mediated glucose uptake, GLUT4 content, and insulin signaling in skeletal muscle in patients with type 2

diabetes. Diabetes. 2004;**53**:294-305. DOI: 10.2337/diabetes.53.2.294

[58] Kuk JL, Kilpatrick K, Davidson LE, Hudson R, Ross R. Whole-body skeletal muscle mass is not related to glucose tolerance or insulin sensitivity in overweight and obese men and women. Applied Physiology, Nutrition, and Metabolism. 2008;**33**:769-774. DOI: 10.1139/H08-060

[59] Hong S, Chang Y, Jung H-S, Yun KE, Shin H, Ryu S. Relative muscle mass and the risk of incident type 2 diabetes: A cohort study. PLoS ONE. 2017;**12**:e0188650. DOI: 10.1371/journal.pone.0188650

[60] Barakat R, Pelaez M, Lopez C, Lucia A, Ruiz JR. Exercise during pregnancy and gestational diabetes-related adverse effects: A randomised controlled trial. British Journal of Sports Medicine. 2013;**47**:630-636. DOI: 10.1136/bjsports-2012-091788

[61] Chu SY, Callaghan WM, Kim SY, Schmid CH, Lau J, England LJ, et al. Maternal obesity and risk of gestational diabetes mellitus. Diabetes Care. 2007;**30**:2070-2076. DOI: 10.2337/dc06-2559a

[62] American Diabetes Association. Management of diabetes in pregnancy: Standards of medical care in diabetes—2018. Diabetes Care. 2018;**41**:S137-S143. DOI: 10.2337/dc18-S013

[63] de Barros MC, Lopes MAB, Francisco RPV, Sapienza AD, Zugaib M. Resistance exercise and glycemic control in women with gestational diabetes mellitus. American Journal of Obstetrics and Gynecology. 2010;**203**:556.e1-556.e6. DOI: 10.1016/j.ajog.2010.07.015

[64] Brankston GN, Mitchell BF, Ryan EA, Okun NB. Resistance exercise decreases the need for insulin in overweight women with gestational diabetes mellitus. American Journal of Obstetrics and Gynecology. 2004;**190**:188-193. DOI: 10.1016/s0002-9378(03)00951-7

[65] Kazemi N, Ali HS. Comparison the effects of aqua aerobic and resistance training on blood sugar and insulin resistance in women with gestational diabetes mellitus. Journal of Physical Activity and Hormones. 2017;**1**:1-18

[66] Kasraeian M, Talebi S, Kazemi N, Bazrafshan K, Asadi N, Idress Ahmad Mohammad R, et al. Insulin resistance and homeostasis model assessment of β-cell function in females with gestational diabetes mellitus: A comparison of aerobic and resistance trainings. Journal of Advanced Medical Sciences and Applied Technologies. 2017;**3**:131-138. DOI: 10.32598/jamsat.3.3.131

[67] Sklempe Kokic I, Ivanisevic M, Kokic T, Simunic B, Pisot R. Acute responses to structured aerobic and resistance exercise in women with gestational diabetes mellitus. Scandinavian Journal of Medicine & Science in Sports. 2018;**28**:1793-1800. DOI: 10.1111/sms.13076

[68] Refaye GEE, Aziz GFA. Comparative study of circuit resistance training and aerobic training on glycemic control of gestational diabetes mellitus. Bulletin of Faculty of Physical Therapy. 2017;**22**:89-95. DOI: 10.4103/bfpt.bfpt_46_16

[69] Stafne SN, Salvesen KÅ, Romundstad PR, Eggebø TM, Carlsen SM, Mørkved S. Regular exercise during pregnancy to prevent gestational diabetes: A randomized controlled trial. Obstetrics & Gynecology. 2012;**119**:29-36. DOI: 10.1097/AOG.0b013e3182393f86

[70] Chevenne D, Trivin F, Porquet D. Insulin assays and reference values.

Diabetes & Metabolism. 1999; **25**:459-476

[71] Reyes-Muñoz E, Martínez-Herrera EM, Ortega-González C, Arce-Sánchez L, Ávila-Carrasco A, Zamora-Escudero R. HOMA-IR and QUICKI reference values during pregnancy in Mexican women. Ginecología y Obstetricia de México. 2017;**85**:306-313

Chapter 6

Pharmacotherapy of Gestational Diabetes Mellitus: Current Recommendations

Miroslav Radenković and Ana Jakovljević

Abstract

The incidence of gestational diabetes mellitus (GDM) is still rising, and this pathological condition is strongly associated with some serious adverse pregnancy outcomes. Therefore, GDM must be timely recognized and adequately managed. Treatment of GDM is aimed to maintain normal glycemia and it should involve regular glucose monitoring, dietary modification, lifestyle changes, moderate physical activity, and pharmacotherapy, when necessary. As for the pharmacotherapy, needed in approximately one-third of GDM women, insulin administration is the first choice of pharmacological treatment, although oral hypoglycemic drugs, for example, metformin (a biguanide agent) or glyburide (a second-generation sulfonylurea drug), could be indicated, too. Metformin is considered as a reasonable and safe first-line alternative to insulin. If comparing two oral agents, metformin seems to be safer than glyburide, since glyburide was found to be linked to neonatal hypoglycemia and higher birth weight, which can for example increase the hazard for shoulder dystocia and a necessity for Cesarean delivery. Finally, it should be underlined that many pregnant women turn to complementary and alternative medicine for health maintenance or symptom relief, including traditional herbal medicine and the use of supplements. Given the previous facts, this chapter will address current pharmacotherapy options and challenges related to GDM treatment.

Keywords: gestational diabetes mellitus, treatment, insulin, metformin, glyburide, oral antidiabetics

1. Introduction

Gestational diabetes mellitus (GDM) is well-described endocrinopathy, referring to any degree of glucose intolerance that develops or else is initially recognized during pregnancy. Today, it is recognized that GDB is most probably a consequence of complex and quite diverse interactions between genetic-epigenetic-environmental factors [1–3]. This diagnosis of gestational diabetes does not include pregnant women who have unrecognized pre-existing diabetes, which today accounts for about 1% of diabetes cases during gestation [4].

GDM is characterized by aberrant fetoplacental vascular function, insulin resistance, and impaired insulin production [5]. Numerous fetal issues have been linked to GDM, for example, macrosomia (birthweight over 4000 g), a higher stillbirth risk, birth trauma, a higher percentage of Cesarean delivery, and newborn hypoglycemia [6]. Most of these have been particularly positively linked to considerable maternal weight fluctuations in GDM [7]. Although today it has become very clear that timely screening and diagnosis (even before 20 weeks gestation) of GDM in at-risk women is more than required for clinically desirable maternal and fetal outcomes [8], in this context, new predictive and diagnostic biomarkers for GDM represent a critical state-of-the-art topic [9].

To circumvent hyperglycemia and its negative effects on fetal growth, pregnant women diagnosed with gestational diabetes are initially managed with individualized medical nutrition therapy and light exercise. Although the majority of scientific associations propose the thresholds for fasting glucose levels of 95 mg/dL and 140 mg/dL at 1-h postprandial, recent findings suggested that decreasing a threshold for blood glucose at 1 h after a meal to less than 120 mg/dL in GDM women lowers the risk of large for gestational age infants and macrosomia, and at the same time without the increased occurrence of small for gestational age infants [10, 11]. This promising finding certainly requires further elucidation.

Insulin has generally been recognized as the first-line drug because it is effective and does not cross the placenta. Other treatment strategies, oral antidiabetic drugs (OAD) such as metformin or glyburide, have been used in recent years given that insulin therapy has several downsides in GDM. Some of them are the absence of a clear dose definition, the need for multiple daily injections, the risk of hypoglycemia, and elevated maternal weight gain [12]. Although oral medications are easy to use and even though they have a high efficacy in the treatment of women with GDM, failure to attain glycemic control appears in around 20% of women, leaving opportunities for new therapeutic optimization [13]. In accordance with previous facts, up-to-date results of available meta-analyses on the effects of antidiabetic pharmaceuticals estimated that if we look to the majority of adverse neonatal outcomes, metformin was ranked to be the superior treatment over insulin or glyburide, whereas the lower risk of adverse maternal outcomes was primarily linked to glyburide administration [14]. These divergent effects require additional caution in their use [8].

Lots of knowledge has been accumulated regarding GDM screening and timely treatment; however, the secondary prevention in women following GDM, as well as in their offspring, represents an important scientific challenge for all of us in many years to come [15].

In this review, we look at how insulin and other oral hypoglycemic medications are used to treat women with GDM, emphasizing on their efficacy and safety. Supplement-related and other alternative pharmacotherapy will be addressed, as well.

2. Current options of pharmacotherapy in GDB

2.1 Insulin and insulin analogs

2.1.1 Pharmacological properties and use

Insulin, due to its huge molecular size, does not pass the placenta unless at extremely high doses [16]. It has a great fetal safety profile; it attains tight maternal glucose control and is therefore recommended as a gold standard, and the first-line treatment for women with GDM. Insulin is not teratogenic, and there is also no evidence that any of them are excreted in human milk [17].

Currently, available insulin analogs are rapidly acting analogs, including aspart and lispro, short-acting regular insulin, intermediate-acting NPH insulin, or longer-acting insulin analogs, such as glargine and detemir [18, 19].

Insulin is the therapy of choice for women who have failed to meet their glycemic treatment goals despite making lifestyle changes—diet and exercise [2]. It can also be used by those who are unable to tolerate the adverse effects of other OADs.

The dose and timing of insulin use are determined by the women's body weight, gestational age, and the time of day when hyperglycemia occurs. Insulin dosage is modified often during pregnancy based on blood glucose values, hypoglycemia, physical activity, nutritional intake, infection, and patient's compliance.

Based on the time of recurrent hyperglycemia, there are two major ways of prescribing insulin. Insulin can be given in divided doses throughout the day or as a single daily dose. Intermediate insulin, such as NPH or detemir, should be given as a single dose at bedtime in GDM women who have hyperglycemia solely in the morning fasting state. Rapid-acting insulin should be administered before a meal in women who have postprandial hyperglycemia. Hyperglycemia during the day should be controlled with a combination of intermediate- or long-acting and short-acting insulin [20].

Close blood glucose monitoring is required while prescribing insulin to avoid hypoglycemia or hyperglycemia. GDM women should bring their self-monitored blood glucose logs to the doctor's office so that the insulin regimen can be adjusted when necessary.

2.1.2 Efficacy and safety

Rapid-acting insulin analogs, often known as bolus insulin, are used to imitate endogenous insulin's response to meal intake. They reach a concentration peak sooner than regular insulin and show a shorter duration of action (3–5 h) [21]. In comparison with human insulin, which must be administered 30 minutes before a meal, rapid-acting insulin analogs can be given 5–10 minutes before a meal, making them more convenient [22]. Basal insulin, also known as intermediate-acting and long-acting insulin, is primarily used to give a constant supply of the modest amounts of insulin to regulate lipolysis and avoid hepatic gluconeogenesis, regardless of meal intake.

Although insulin treatment has traditionally been the drug of choice for treating hyperglycemia in GDM after medical nutrition and physical exercise, it is not without limitations. Many pregnant women face issues with insulin administration, including gaining weight, balancing dosage, diet, and, for some, the frequency of hypoglycemic episodes. For that reason, there are quite a few reports currently suggesting metformin as the first-line agent having an equivalent efficacy *vs.* insulin, yet with less hypoglycemia than insulin [23].

Short-acting insulin has been connected to an augmented risk of hypoglycemia and glycemic control changes in those with GDM. Aspart's recent experience has been positive, although lispro has been linked to higher birth weight and a greater rate of large for gestational age newborns [24]. In randomized clinical investigations comparing detemir to NPH for intermediate- and longer-acting insulin, there was no difference in glucose management or perinatal outcomes. Detemir has been linked to a lower risk of hypoglycemia in diabetics who are not pregnant [25].

2.2 Oral antihyperglycemic drugs (OAD)

2.2.1 Metformin

2.2.1.1 Pharmacological properties and use

Metformin, an oral biguanide, works by reducing liver gluconeogenesis, increasing peripheral insulin sensitivity, and also promoting glucose uptake in peripheral tissues while lowering glucose absorption in the gut [26]. Several mechanisms are responsible for higher insulin sensitivity including the augmented activity of insulin receptor tyrosine kinase, enhanced synthesis of glycogen, reduction of glycogenolysis, decreased activity of hepatic glucose-6-phosphatase, and an increase in the recruitment and activity of GLUT4 glucose transporters [27]. It decreases fasting serum insulin by 40% (thus lowers the risk of hypoglycemia) and leads to a 5.8% weight loss on average [28]. Despite identical glycemic control, metformin was related to lower cardiovascular, as well as all-cause mortality if paralleled to sulphonylureas and insulin in a long-term prospective study of type 2 diabetes. The RISK pathway activation *via* increased AMPK activity may be responsible for this effect [29, 30].

Organic cation transporters (OCTs) transport metformin across the mitochondrial membrane at the cellular level. Since the placenta expresses many OCT isoforms, metformin crosses the placenta easily during pregnancy. Concerns about potential negative effects on fetal development arise from transport *via* the placenta into the developing fetus. Although it is unknown if OCTs are expressed in human embryos, we know that pre-implantation human embryos have limited mitochondrial capacity making them resistant to metformin [31, 32]. In Metformin in gestational diabetes study (MiG), children (aged 2) exposed to metformin during pregnancy were compared to children of the same age whose mothers were on insulin during pregnancy. Children exposed to metformin had comparable overall body fat, yet more subcutaneous fat over intra-abdominal fat compared to children exposed to insulin, thus suggesting that metformin treatment may lead to a more advantageous pattern of fat distribution than insulin [33].

Only recently there has been evidence to support the use of metformin for the management of GDM. It has, however, been used in early pregnancy and all through pregnancy for additional indications for decades. Metformin can help women with the polycystic ovarian syndrome to establish regular ovulation and to enhance conceiving odds, and by using it during the first trimester to lower the incidence of spontaneous abortion [34]. Metformin's use and effectiveness in the management of insulin-dependent T2DM in pregnancy have been supported by early research [35]. Despite this, it was not until the metformin in Gestational Diabetes trial, presented by Rowan et al. in 2008, was widely reported as an effective treatment for GDM [36].

2.2.1.2 Efficacy and safety

In the gestational diabetes trial [36], women were randomly assigned to either metformin or standard treatment, that is, insulin. Supplemental insulin was required by a large percentage of women using metformin (46%), however at much lower doses than GDM-women using insulin as monotherapy. The key outcome was a combination of neonatal hypoglycemia (2.6 mmol/L), respiratory distress, requirement for phototherapy, 5-minute Apgar score of 7, or premature birth (before 37 weeks), and it was similar in both treatment groups. Women who took metformin gained considerably less weight from enrolment to term than those who took insulin. Other parameters considered in the metformin and insulin clusters were similar, including birth weight, neonatal anthropometrics, and odds for large for gestational age. However, when compared to insulin therapy, the incidence of severe hypoglycemia (1.6 mmol/L) was lower in the metformin group. This research also discovered that patient acceptability for metformin was substantially better than with insulin; when questioned if they would select it yet again for future pregnancies, 77 percent of metformin users replied yes, compared to only 27 percent of insulin users. Metformin's gastrointestinal side effects caused 32 women (8.8%) to cut their dose, although only 7 (1.9%) had to discontinue taking it.

A group of 100 GDM women merely treated with metformin *vs.* 100 women with GDM only treated with insulin were matched for age, weight, and ethnicity in a case–control observational study [37]. Maternal risk factors were similar in both groups. The rates of preeclampsia, prenatal hypertension, and Cesarean section were identical, but an average maternal gain of weight from enrolment to term was considerably lower in the metformin group, just as it was in the MiG study. When compared to women who were treated with insulin, women who were given metformin had a lower rate of preterm, neonatal jaundice, and admission to a neonatal unit, as well as an overall improvement in newborn morbidity [37].

Post-prandial glycemic levels may indeed be of importance when comparing metformin to other treatment options. A meta-analysis of three randomized controlled studies of GDM women found lower post-prandial glucose in metformin as opposed to insulin-treated patients, though these disparities did not meet statistical significance [38].

Metformin did not raise the risk of preterm delivery or Cesarean section, as reported in a latest systematic review, nor did it raise the risk of small for gestational age newborns. Metformin, on the other hand, was linked to a lower risk of preterm birth, newborn hypoglycemia, and admission to neonatal intensive care units, as well as a decreased prevalence of pregnancy-induced hypertension [39].

Because metformin is not stimulating the secretion of insulin, it does not provoke maternal hypoglycemia, which is a side effect that remains a concern with glyburide. For the same reason, severe neonatal hypoglycemia is less likely to occur after metformin administration compared to insulin [14]. Accordingly, hypoglycemia is a greater risk if taking insulin, than with OAD [40]. Metformin, on the other hand, crosses the placental barrier easily due to its low molecular mass, hydrophilic nature, and lack of protein binding [41]. Metformin concentrations in the fetus are likely minimal and no fetal side effects, such as congenital malformations, have been detected [42]. It is not thought to be teratogenic, as evidenced by decades of use in preconception and early pregnancy. There have been no reports of newborn lactic acidosis, and neonatal hypoglycemia has been related to maternal hyperglycemia during delivery rather than a direct side effect of metformin. It belongs to the FDA's Pregnancy Category B.

Before starting metformin treatment, patients should be informed about the potential for maternal adverse effects. Although its mechanism of action does not produce hypoglycemia directly, symptoms are observed in 0–10% of women who administered the drug. A 5 percent to 15% of women experienced gastrointestinal side effects, such as flatulence, nausea, diarrhea, and vomiting. Lactic acidosis, the most worrying potential side effect, was prevented by gradually raising the dose [43].

One final question could be certainly related to the eventual advantageous co-administration of metformin and insulin in GDM. Scarce reports have been published over the past decade; however, Chaves et al. [44] recently addressed this issue through the retrospective investigation with an evaluation of the Portuguese National Registry of GDM (2012–2017) with a very interesting report that in GDM women the concomitant use of metformin and insulin resulted in comparable obstetric and neonatal adverse events if paralleled with insulin monotherapy. Moreover, the authors reported that expected beneficial effects on weight gain and insulin dose were simply not detected if both drugs were used in a parallel manner [44].

2.2.2 Glyburide

2.2.2.1 Pharmacological properties and use

Glyburide is a second-generation sulfonylurea that acts mainly by increasing the secretion of insulin from the pancreas and improving the insulin sensitivity of peripheral tissues. These actions can be detected after a block of the sulfonylurea receptor, which is actually a part of the ATP-sensitive potassium channel in the pancreatic beta cells [45]. Glyburide is lipophilic and significantly bound to albumin [46].

At first, it was assumed that glyburide did not cross the placenta. Langer et al. (2000) did not detect glyburide in umbilical cord serum of neonates whose mothers were taking glyburide during pregnancy, thus confirming *in vitro* investigations that found no glyburide transfer in-between mother and fetus. The reason behind that is that they used liquid chromatography with a limit of detection of 10 ng per milliliter [13]. Newer studies proved that glyburide can be found in umbilical cord serum by using a highly sensitive liquid chromatography-mass spectrometry test for determining glyburide at sub-ng/mL levels, confirming that glyburide is actually transferred transplacentally [47].

There is an obvious option to glyburide and that is insulin administration. Even though glyburide is an FDA category C drug, compared to insulin analogs (lispro, detemir, and aspart) that are all pregnancy risk factor B medications, glyburide is still widely used. The situation where glyburide is a better choice is where self-monitoring of glucose blood levels needed for insulin or insulin storage is not possible or where a patient has a severe needle phobia.

Another benefit of using glyburide is that it is a low-cost oral agent, easy to take with few side effects. Also, glyburide is, as an oral agent just like metformin, easier to use compared to insulin [41]. Nevertheless, the other use of glyburide during pregnancy for GDM patients is still unclear and needs to be comprehensively elucidated [48].

2.2.2.2 Efficacy and safety

The New England Journal of Medicine published a clinical investigation comparing glyburide versus insulin in management of GDM in 2000, which transformed the management of GDM. Namely, Langer et al. (2000) conducted the first randomized, controlled study where they compared glyburide to insulin by dividing 404 women with GDM into two groups, 201 receiving glyburide and 203 receiving insulin [49]. Results did not show any significant difference between the two clusters in neonatal outcomes by measuring high blood glucose concentrations, the incidence of macrosomia, admission to neonatal intensive care unit, etc. The authors also noted that the extent of glycemic control between the two groups was similar. A different study comparing macrosomia, neonatal hypoglycemia, and hyperbilirubinemia in two groups found no evidence that using glyburide instead of subcutaneous insulin leads to a higher rate of perinatal problems [50]. On the contrary, a retrospective cohort study analyzed data from 9173 women diagnosed with GDM and treated with glyburide opposite to insulin 150 days before delivery [37]. It was found that newborns delivered by women treated with glyburide were more expected to have complications than those delivered by mothers who were taking insulin. Complications noted were preterm birth, Cesarean delivery, hypoglycemia, respiratory distress, jaundice, birth injury, large for gestational age, and hospitalization in the neonatal ICU [51].

Seven trials comparing glyburide (n = 457) to insulin (n = 467) were analyzed in one more recent meta-analyses by Jiang et al. to assess the efficacy and safety of oral anti-diabetic (OADs) medicines for GDM. In terms of glycemic management, the investigators did not find any difference between glyburide and insulin. Glyburide therapy, on the other hand, is linked to a higher risk of neonatal hypoglycemia, high neonatal birth weight, high maternal weight gain, and macrosomia [52].

A group of 457 glyburide-managed pregnancies and 467 insulin-treated pregnancies were evaluated in the Jiang meta-analysis comparing the efficacy and safety of OAD for GDM [52]. Despite no dissimilarity in glycemic control, the authors found that glyburide caused considerably more macrosomia than insulin (OR: 3.09, 95% CI: 1.59–6.04, P = 0.009). Glyburide was also associated with a greater rate of newborn hypoglycemia than insulin (OR: 2.64, 95% CI: 1.59–4.28, P = 0.0002). There was no difference in weight growth, Cesarean delivery rate, or preeclampsia between NICU admissions or premature births.

Finally, it has to be underlined that glyburide was ranked the worst in the recent meta-analysis, with the highest rates of macrosomia, hyperbilirubinemia, preeclampsia, neonatal hypoglycemia, low birth weight, preterm birth, and metformin (plus insulin when needed) had the lowest rates of pregnancy hypertension, macrosomia, LGA, RDS, preterm birth, and low birth weight [53]. Besides, one has to be very cautious with glyburide use, which was shown to be associated with weight gain, as well as maternal hypoglycemia, especially when taken without any food [45].

2.2.3 Acarbose

2.2.3.1 Pharmacological properties and use

Acarbose is an alpha-glucosidase inhibitor, which means it prevents enzymes found on the small intestine's brush border from breaking down complex starches into oligosaccharides and oligosaccharides, trisaccharides, and disaccharides into glucose. As a result, the rise in postprandial glucose concentrations is lowered. Its use is usually linked to gastrointestinal complications. Although just 2% of acarbose is absorbed as an active medication, 34% of its metabolites were found in the systemic circulation [54].

Acarbose is not usually recommended for the treatment of GDM, because it has not been thoroughly researched during pregnancy and considering safer and more acceptable options, with more information regarding treating GDM, such as insulin and metformin.

2.2.3.2 Efficacy and safety

One small randomized prospective study (n = 70) in Brazil compared glyburide and acarbose to insulin in the treatment of GDM and showed the absence of notable differences in fasting or postprandial glucose concentrations with acarbose, although gastrointestinal side effects were higher in occurrence with acarbose [55]. Acarbose showed a higher failure rate (42%) in establishing glycemic control compared to glyburide (21%). Neonatal hypoglycemia occurred in one acarbose-treated subject, one insulin-treated subject, and eight glyburide-treated subjects. Only four neonates (16%) developed macrosomia, which is after receiving glyburide therapy.

Although in this short trial, failure to achieve glycemic control with acarbose was higher if compared to glyburide, the decreased incidence of hypoglycemia and macrosomia underlines acarbose as an appealing agent to investigate in future GDM treatment studies. Accordingly, in the recent investigation published by Jayasingh et al. (2020), it was proposed that acarbose can be seen as an effective and adequately tolerated choice for the management of GDM [56]. Namely, this prospective, open-label, and controlled study was designed to compare the fetomaternal outcomes in pregnant women with GDM designated to insulin or acarbose group. Thus, no difference was found if the following parameters were paralleled in between the groups: the incidence of recurrent infections, preeclampsia, or premature rupture of membranes; then the modes of delivery, mean postoperative random blood glucose, fasting blood glucose level at day 7 and after 6 weeks; and finally difference in the mean birth weight of offspring born to mothers treated with either of the two pharmacological agents.

Even though using acarbose in diabetic patients has been linked to abnormal liver enzymes and hepatic failure, a newer study did not show a higher risk of liver injury during acarbose treatment [57]. Acarbose can pass through the placenta. In pregnant animal investigations, doses up to 32 times higher than the human dose were not proven to be teratogenic. On the other hand, it induces stomach cramps and may raise prostaglandin E, suggesting that it possess the potential ability to induce labor [58].

3. Supplementation and traditional treatment options

The efficacy of vitamin and mineral supplementation in GDM patients is still under investigation. However, today is known that in GDM, low levels of vitamin D, vitamin E, and magnesium have been detected, whereas glucose metabolism, anti-inflammatory, and anti-oxidative stress have been all positively regulated after vitamin D, vitamin E, magnesium, and selenium supplementation, which was also confirmed in the very recent meta-analysis reported by Li et al. [59]. In the same manner, 6-week-long Mg-Zn-Ca-vitamin D co-supplementation reduced biomarkers of inflammation and oxidative stress in GDM women [60]. To continue, the improvement in glycemic control and decline of adverse fetomaternal outcomes after vitamin D supplementation (including Cesarean section, postpartum hemorrhage, maternal hospitalization, neonatal hyperbilirubinemia, giant children, fetal distress, polyhydramnios, premature delivery) was underlined by Wang et al. [61].

Dietary adjustments accompanied with lifestyle modifications are known to achieve normoglycemia in a majority of women with GDM, especially underlining careful attention to type and amount of dietary carbohydrates [62]. In this context, myoinositol, a dietary supplement knowing to decrease insulin resistance, became extensively investigated [63]. It represents inositol isomer organically present for example in legumes or nuts, but also synthesized in kidneys and liver to a certain extent. Accordingly, recent findings pointed out that, if started shortly after the GDM diagnosis, myoinositol (1000 mg twice daily, *per os*) was shown to be effective in reaching glycemic control and reducing the need for additional pharmacotherapy [64].

Traditional Chinese medicine and herbal products, known to be broadly utilized during human history, now belong to a very interesting field currently investigated in the frame of GDM [65]. So far, herbs such as *Zuo Gui Wan*, red raspberry tea, and *Orthosiphon stamineus* all provided valid possibilities in reducing glucose and alleviating the GDM-related pathophysiology, and at the same time with good safety profile to the mother and neonate [66]. In addition, the antidiabetic potential of glycyrrhiza flavonoids from traditional Chinese medicine, as adjuvants for insulin therapy, could be especially beneficial in GDM [67].

Finally, probiotics supplementation in improving glycemic control and attenuating some of the adverse events related to GDM is a very interesting and appealing scientific issue that needs further elucidation [68, 69].

Even though new and promising results are published every day, novel investigations and, most of all, well-designed standardized protocols are needed for obtaining original, comparable, and sustainable results in this field of adjuvant GDM treatment.

4. Conclusions

In the twenty-first century, GDM poses a significant challenge to health care professionals. The short- and long-term effects of successfully controlling GDM are important for both the mother and the fetus. This chapter provided data related to proposed pharmacological treatment options for GDM, further evaluating each therapy's unique characteristics, benefits, and drawbacks in comparison with the alternatives. Most guidelines recommend oral pharmacological therapy, such as glyburide and metformin, and it is now widely used, with data on efficacy and safety. They can both be used as the first-line option; however, metformin appears to be preferable to glyburide in terms of newborn and maternal outcomes, while it is associated with a higher incidence of failure to achieve appropriate glycemic control. Analogs such as detemir, aspart, and lispro, which have been thoroughly proved for their safety and efficacy during pregnancy, are indicated as first-line therapy or when oral medication fails to achieve optimal glucose control. Glargine can be used during pregnancy, while there is not as much data to back it up as there is for other long-acting analogs and human insulins.

Therefore, the pharmacological treatment for GDM should be adapted to the patient's characteristics, glycemic profile, and preferences, as well as local professional body guidelines. While insulin has typically been used to treat GDM, both metformin and glyburide may be used, but patients should be informed about the risks and advantages.

Pharmacotherapy of GDM is still under investigation, even though much is known about GDB itself. We can witness that the molecular understanding of GMB has been constantly translated to more efficacious and safer therapeutic options. Still, we expect that coordinated and well-focused basic and clinical investigations will provide even more precise information regarding future choices for prevention and adequate, as well as timely treatment of GDM.

Author details

Miroslav Radenković* and Ana Jakovljević
Faculty of Medicine, Department of Pharmacology, Clinical Pharmacology and Toxicology, University of Belgrade, Serbia

*Address all correspondence to: miroslav.radenkovic@med.bg.ac.rs

References

[1] Rosik J, Szostak B, Machaj F, Pawlik A. The role of genetics and epigenetics in the pathogenesis of gestational diabetes mellitus. Annals of Human Genetics. 2020;**84**(2):114-124. DOI: 10.1111/ahg.12356

[2] McIntyre HD, Catalano P, Zhang C, Desoye G, Mathiesen ER, Damm P. Gestational diabetes mellitus. Nature Reviews. Disease Primers. 2019;**5**(1):47. DOI: 10.1038/s41572-019-0098-8

[3] Franzago M, Fraticelli F, Stuppia L, Vitacolonna E. Nutrigenetics, epigenetics and gestational diabetes: Consequences in mother and child. Epigenetics. 2019;**14**(3):215-235. DOI: 10.1080/15592294.2019.1582277

[4] Radenkovic M. Treatment considerations for gestational diabetes mellitus and long-term postpartum options. In: Gestational Diabetes. IntechOpen; 2011. pp. 315-324. DOI: 10.5772/21908

[5] Subiabre M, Silva L, Toledo F, Paublo M, López MA, Boric MP, et al. Insulin therapy and its consequences for the mother, foetus, and newborn in gestational diabetes mellitus. Biochimica et Biophysica Acta - Molecular Basis of Disease. 2018;**1864** (9 Pt B):2949-2956. DOI: 10.1016/j.bbadis.2018.06.005

[6] Singh KP, Rahimpanah F, Barclay M. Metformin for the management of gestational diabetes mellitus. The Australian & New Zealand Journal of Obstetrics & Gynaecology. 2015;**55**(4):303-308. DOI: 10.1111/ajo.12311

[7] Gou BH, Guan HM, Bi YX, Ding BJ. Gestational diabetes: Weight gain during pregnancy and its relationship to pregnancy outcomes. Chinese Medical Journal. 2019;**132**(2):154-160. DOI: 10.1097/CM9.0000000000000036

[8] Mirabelli M, Chiefari E, Tocci V, Greco E, Foti D, Brunetti A. Gestational diabetes: Implications for fetal growth, intervention timing, and treatment options. Current Opinion in Pharmacology. 2021;**60**:1-10. DOI: 10.1016/j.coph.2021.06.003

[9] Lorenzo-Almorós A, Hang T, Peiró C, Soriano-Guillén L, Egido J, Tuñón J, et al. Predictive and diagnostic biomarkers for gestational diabetes and its associated metabolic and cardiovascular diseases. Cardiovascular Diabetology. 2019;**18**(1):140. DOI: 10.1186/s12933-019-0935-9

[10] Szmuilowicz ED, Josefson JL, Metzger BE. Gestational diabetes mellitus. Endocrinology and Metabolism Clinics of North America. 2019;**48**(3):479-493. DOI: 10.1016/j.ecl.2019.05.001

[11] Żurawska-Kliś M, Czarnik K, Szymczak S, Wójcik M, Cypryk K. 1-Hour postprandial glucose target of < 120 mg/dL is superior to < 140 mg/dL in the treatment for gestational diabetes mellitus in relation to pregnancy outcomes: A retrospective study. Acta Diabetologica. 2021;**58**(5):665-668. DOI: 10.1007/s00592-020-01655-w

[12] Norman RJ, Wang JX, Hague W. Should we continue or stop insulin sensitizing drugs during pregnancy? Current Opinion in Obstetrics & Gynecology. 2004;**16**(3):245-250. DOI: 10.1097/00001703-200406000-00007

[13] Langer O, Conway DL, Berkus MD, Xenakis EM, Gonzales O. A comparison of glyburide and insulin in women with gestational diabetes mellitus. The New England Journal of Medicine. 2000;**343**(16):1134-1138. DOI: 10.1056/NEJM200010193431601

[14] Bidhendi Yarandi R, Amiri M, Ramezani Tehrani F,

Behboudi-Gandevani S. Effectiveness of antidiabetic agents for treatment of gestational diabetes: A methodological quality assessment of meta-analyses and NETWORK META-ANALYSIS. Journal of Diabetes Investigation. 2021. DOI: 10.1111/jdi.13603

[15] Sheiner E. Gestational diabetes mellitus: Long-term consequences for the mother and child grand challenge: How to move on towards secondary prevention? Frontiers in Clinical Diabetes and Healthcare. 2020;**1**:1. DOI: 10.3389/fcdhc.2020.546256

[16] Challier JC, Hauguel S, Desmaizieres V. Effect of insulin on glucose uptake and metabolism in the human placenta. The Journal of Clinical Endocrinology and Metabolism. 1986;**62**(5):803-807. DOI: 10.1210/jcem-62-5-803

[17] Martis R, Crowther CA, Shepherd E, Alsweiler J, Downie MR, Brown J. Treatments for women with gestational diabetes mellitus: An overview of Cochrane systematic reviews. Cochrane Database of Systematic Reviews. 2018;**8**:CD012327. DOI: 10.1002/14651858.CD012327.pub2

[18] Lende M, Rijhsinghani A. Gestational diabetes: Overview with emphasis on medical management. International Journal of Environmental Research and Public Health. 2020;**17**(24):9573. DOI: 10.3390/ijerph17249573

[19] Kautzky-Willer A, Harreiter J, Winhofer-Stöckl Y, Bancher-Todesca D, Berger A, Repa A, et al. Gestational diabetes mellitus (Update 2019). Wiener Klinische Wochenschrift. 2019;**131**(Suppl 1):91-102. DOI: 10.1007/s00508-018-1419-8

[20] Committee on Practice Bulletins-Obstetrics. ACOG practice bulletin no. 190: Gestational diabetes mellitus. Obstetrics and Gynecology. 2018;**131**(2):e49-e64. DOI: 10.1097/AOG.0000000000002501

[21] Toledano Y, Hadar E, Hod M. Safety of insulin analogues as compared with human insulin in pregnancy. Expert Opinion on Drug Safety. 2016;**15**(7):963-973. DOI: 10.1080/14740338.2016.1182153

[22] Pettitt DJ, Ospina P, Kolaczynski JW, Jovanovic L. Comparison of an insulin analog, insulin aspart, and regular human insulin with no insulin in gestational diabetes mellitus. Diabetes Care. 2003;**26**(1):183-186. DOI: 10.2337/diacare.26.1.183

[23] Musa OAH, Syed A, Mohamed AM, Chivese T, Clark J, Furuya-Kanamori L, et al. Metformin is comparable to insulin for pharmacotherapy in gestational diabetes mellitus: A network meta-analysis evaluating 6046 women. Pharmacological Research. 2021;**167**(105546):105546. DOI: 10.1016/j.phrs.2021.105546

[24] Lv S, Wang J, Xu Y. Safety of insulin analogs during pregnancy: A meta-analysis. Archives of Gynecology and Obstetrics. 2015;**292**(4):749-756. DOI: 10.1007/s00404-015-3692-3

[25] Herrera KM, Rosenn BM, Foroutan J, Bimson BE, Al Ibraheemi Z, Moshier EL, et al. Randomized controlled trial of insulin detemir versus NPH for the treatment of pregnant women with diabetes. American Journal of Obstetrics and Gynecology. 2015;**213**(3):426.e1-426.e7. DOI: 10.1016/j.ajog.2015.06.010

[26] Scarpello JHB, Howlett HCS. Metformin therapy and clinical uses. Diabetes & Vascular Disease Research. 2008;**5**(3):157-167. DOI: 10.3132/dvdr.2008.027

[27] Wiernsperger NF, Bailey CJ. The antihyperglycaemic effect of metformin: Therapeutic and cellular mechanisms.

Drugs. 1999;**58**(Supplement 1):31-39. DOI: 10.2165/00003495-199958001-00009

[28] Glueck CJ, Goldenberg N, Wang P, Loftspring M, Sherman A. Metformin during pregnancy reduces insulin, insulin resistance, insulin secretion, weight, testosterone and development of gestational diabetes: Prospective longitudinal assessment of women with polycystic ovary syndrome from preconception throughout pregnancy. Human Reproduction. 2004;**19**(3):510-521. DOI: 10.1093/humrep/deh109

[29] King P, Peacock I, Donnelly R. The UK prospective diabetes study (UKPDS): Clinical and therapeutic implications for type 2 diabetes: Therapeutic implications of the UKPDS. British Journal of Clinical Pharmacology. 1999;**48**(5):643-648. DOI: 10.1046/j.1365-2125.1999.00092.x

[30] Giannarelli R, Aragona M, Coppelli A, Del Prato S. Reducing insulin resistance with metformin: The evidence today. Diabetes & Metabolism. 2003;**29**(4):6S28-6S35. DOI: 10.1016/s1262-3636(03)72785-2

[31] Ahmadimoghaddam D, Hofman J, Zemankova L, Nachtigal P, Dolezelova E, Cerveny L, et al. Synchronized activity of organic cation transporter 3 (Oct3/Slc22a3) and multidrug and toxin extrusion 1 (Mate1/Slc47a1) transporter in transplacental passage of MPP+ in rat. Toxicological Sciences. 2012;**128**(2):471-481. DOI: 10.1093/toxsci/kfs160

[32] Cho YM, Kwon S, Pak YK, Seol HW, Choi YM, Park DJ, et al. Dynamic changes in mitochondrial biogenesis and antioxidant enzymes during the spontaneous differentiation of human embryonic stem cells. Biochemical and Biophysical Research Communications. 2006;**348**(4):1472-1478. DOI: 10.1016/j.bbrc.2006.08.020

[33] Rowan JA, Rush EC, Obolonkin V, Battin M, Wouldes T, Hague WM. Metformin in gestational diabetes: The offspring follow-up (MiG TOFU): Body composition at 2 years of age. Diabetes Care. 2011;**34**(10):2279-2284. DOI: 10.2337/dc11-0660

[34] Kumar P, Khan K. Effects of metformin use in pregnant patients with polycystic ovary syndrome. Journal of Human Reproductive Sciences. 2012;**5**(2):166. DOI: 10.4103/0974-1208.101012

[35] Rowan JA, Hague WM, Gao W, Battin MR, Moore MP. Metformin versus insulin for the treatment of gestational diabetes. New England Journal of Medicine. 2008;**358**(19):2003-2015. DOI: 10.1056/NEJMoa0707193

[36] Balani J, Hyer SL, Rodin DA, Shehata H. Pregnancy outcomes in women with gestational diabetes treated with metformin or insulin: A case-control study. Diabetic Medicine. 2009;**26**(8):798-802. DOI: 10.1111/j.1464-5491.2009.02780.x

[37] Gui J, Liu Q, Feng L. Metformin vs insulin in the management of gestational diabetes: A meta-analysis. PLoS ONE. 2013;**8**(5):e64585. DOI: 10.1371/journal.pone.0064585

[38] Butalia S, Gutierrez L, Lodha A, Aitken E, Zakariasen A, Donovan L. Short- and long-term outcomes of metformin compared with insulin alone in pregnancy: A systematic review and meta-analysis. Diabetic Medicine. 2016;**34**(1):27-36. DOI: 10.1111/dme.13150

[39] Berggren ERICAK, Boggess KIMA. Oral agents for the management of gestational diabetes. Clinical Obstetrics and Gynecology. 2013;**56**(4):827-836. DOI: 10.1097/GRF.0b013e3182a8e0a5

[40] Charles B, Norris R, Xiao X, Hague W. Population pharmacokinetics

of metformin in late pregnancy. Therapeutic Drug Monitoring. 2006;**28**(1):67-72. DOI: 10.1097/01.ftd.0000184161.52573.0e

[41] Vanky E, Zahlsen K, Spigset O, Carlsen S. Placental passage of metformin in women with polycystic ovary syndrome. Fertility and Sterility. 2005;**83**(5):1575-1578. DOI: 10.1016/j.fertnstert.2004.11.051

[42] Gilbert C, Valois M, Koren G. Pregnancy outcome after first-trimester exposure to metformin: A meta-analysis. Fertility and Sterility. 2006;**86**(3):658-663. DOI: 10.1016/j.fertnstert.2006.02.098

[43] Bolen S, Feldman L, Vassy J, Wilson L, Yeh HC, Marinopoulos S, et al. Systematic review: Comparative effectiveness and safety of oral medications for type 2 diabetes mellitus. Annals of Internal Medicine. 2007;**147**(6):386. DOI: 10.7326/0003-4819-147-6-200709180-00178

[44] Chaves C, Cunha F, Martinho M, Garrido S, Silva-Vieira M, Estevinho C, et al. Metformin combined with insulin in women with gestational diabetes mellitus: A propensity score-matched study. Acta Diabetologica. 2021;**58**(5):615-621. DOI: 10.1007/s00592-020-01665-8

[45] Blair RA, Rosenberg EA, Palermo NE. The use of non-insulin agents in gestational diabetes: Clinical considerations in tailoring therapy. Current Diabetes Reports. 2019;**19**(12):158. DOI: 10.1007/s11892-019-1243-1

[46] Malek R, Davis SN. Pharmacokinetics, efficacy and safety of glyburide for treatment of gestational diabetes mellitus. Expert Opinion on Drug Metabolism & Toxicology. 2016;**12**(6):691-699. DOI: 10.1080/17425255.2016.1187131

[47] Naraharisetti S, Kirby B, Hebert M, Easterling T, Unadkat J. Validation of a sensitive LC–MS assay for quantification of glyburide and its metabolite 4-transhydroxy glyburide in plasma and urine: An OPRU Network study. Journal of Chromatography B. 2007;**860**(1):34-41. DOI: 10.1002/bmc.3314

[48] Guo L, Ma J, Tang J, Hu D, Zhang W, Zhao X. Comparative efficacy and safety of metformin, glyburide, and insulin in treating gestational diabetes mellitus: A meta-analysis. Journal Diabetes Research. 2019;**2019**:9804708. DOI: 10.1155/2019/9804708

[49] Langer O, Yogev Y, Xenakis EMJ, Rosenn B. Insulin and glyburide therapy: Dosage, severity level of gestational diabetes, and pregnancy outcome. American Journal of Obstetrics and Gynecology. 2005;**192**(1):134-139. DOI: 10.1016/j.ajog.2004.07.011

[50] Sénat MV, Affres H, Letourneau A, Coustols-Valat M, Cazaubiel M, Legardeur H, et al. Effect of glyburide vs subcutaneous insulin on perinatal complications among women with gestational diabetes. JAMA. 2018;**319**(17):1773. DOI: 10.1001/jama.2018.4072

[51] Camelo Castillo W, Boggess K, Stürmer T, Brookhart MA, Benjamin DK, Jonsson Funk M. Association of adverse pregnancy outcomes with glyburide vs insulin in women with gestational diabetes. JAMA Pediatrics. 2015;**169**(5):452. DOI: 10.1001/jamapediatrics.2015.74

[52] Jiang YF, Chen XY, Ding T, Wang XF, Zhu ZN, Su SW. Comparative efficacy and safety of OADs in management of GDM: Network meta-analysis of randomized controlled trials. The Journal of Clinical Endocrinology & Metabolism. 2015;**100**(5):2071-2080. DOI: 10.1210/jc.2014-4403

[53] H-Ling L, S-Juan M, Y-Ni X, H-Zhuan T. Comparative efficacy and safety of oral antidiabetic drugs and insulin in treating gestational diabetes mellitus. Medicine (Baltimore). 2017;**96**(38):e7939. DOI: 10.1097/MD.0000000000007939

[54] Simmons D. Safety considerations with pharmacological treatment of gestational diabetes mellitus. Drug Safety. 2014;**38**(1):65-78. DOI: 10.1007/s40264-014-0253-9

[55] Bertini AM, Silva JC, Taborda W, Becker F, Bebber FR, Viesi JM, et al. Perinatal outcomes and the use of oral hypoglycemic agents. Journal of Perinatal Medicine. 2005;**33**(6):519-23. DOI: 10.1515/JPM.2005.092

[56] Jayasingh S Sr, Nanda S, Misra S, Baliarsinha A, Das S, Patil A. Comparison of fetomaternal outcomes in patients with gestational diabetes mellitus treated with insulin versus acarbose: Results of a prospective, open label, controlled study. Cureus. 2020;**12**(12):e12283. DOI: 10.7759/cureus.12283

[57] Chao CT, Wang J, Huang JW, Chien KL. Acarbose use and liver injury in diabetic patients with severe renal insufficiency and hepatic diseases: A propensity score-matched cohort study. Frontiers in Pharmacology. 2018;**9**:860. DOI: 10.3389/fphar.2018.00860

[58] Singh AK, Singh R. Oral antidiabetic agents in gestational diabetes: A narrative review of current evidence. Expert Review of Endocrinology and Metabolism. 2014;**10**(2):211-225. DOI: 10.1586/17446651.2015.982090

[59] Li D, Cai Z, Pan Z, Yang Y, Zhang J. The effects of vitamin and mineral supplementation on women with gestational diabetes mellitus. BMC Endocrine Disorders. 2021;**21**(1):106. DOI: 10.1186/s12902-021-00712-x

[60] Jamilian M, Mirhosseini N, Eslahi M, Bahmani F, Shokrpour M, Chamani M, et al. The effects of magnesium-zinc-calcium-vitamin D co-supplementation on biomarkers of inflammation, oxidative stress and pregnancy outcomes in gestational diabetes. BMC Pregnancy and Childbirth. 2019;**19**(1):107. DOI: 10.1186/s12884-019-2258-y

[61] Wang M, Chen Z, Hu Y, Wang Y, Wu Y, Lian F, et al. The effects of vitamin D supplementation on glycemic control and maternal-neonatal outcomes in women with established gestational diabetes mellitus: A systematic review and meta-analysis. Clinical Nutrition. 2021;**40**(5):3148-3157. DOI: 10.1016/j.clnu.2020.12.016

[62] Mustad VA, Huynh DTT, López-Pedrosa JM, Campoy C, Rueda R. The role of dietary carbohydrates in gestational diabetes. Nutrients. 2020;**12**(2):385. DOI: 10.3390/nu12020385

[63] D'Anna R, Santamaria A, Alibrandi A, Corrado F, DI Benedetto A, Facchinetti F. Myo-inositol for the prevention of gestational diabetes mellitus. A brief review. Journal of Nutritional Science and Vitaminology (Tokyo). 2019;**65**(Supplement):S59-S61. DOI: 10.3177/jnsv.65.S59

[64] Kulshrestha V, Balani S, Kachhawa G, Vanamail P, Kumari R, Sharma JB, et al. Efficacy of myoinositol in treatment of gestational diabetes mellitus in Asian Indian women: A pilot randomized clinical trial. European Journal of Obstetrics, Gynecology, and Reproductive Biology. 2021;**260**:42-47. DOI: 10.1016/j.ejogrb.2021.02.017

[65] Wang CC, Li L, Shao YF, Liu XK, Tam WH, Li RM. Chinese herbal medicines for treating gestational

diabetes mellitus. Cochrane Database Syst Rev. 2019(6):CD013354. DOI:10.1002/14651858.CD013354

[66] Xu YXZ, Xi S, Qian X. Evaluating traditional Chinese medicine and herbal products for the treatment of gestational diabetes mellitus. Journal Diabetes Research. 2019;**2019**:9182595. DOI: 10.1155/2019/9182595

[67] Bai L, Li X, He L, Zheng Y, Lu H, Li J, et al. Antidiabetic potential of flavonoids from traditional Chinese medicine: A review. The American Journal of Chinese Medicine. 2019;**47**(5):933-957. DOI: 10.1142/S0192415X19500496

[68] Zhang J, Ma S, Wu S, Guo C, Long S, Tan H. Effects of probiotic supplement in pregnant women with gestational diabetes mellitus: A systematic review and meta-analysis of randomized controlled trials. Journal Diabetes Research. 2019;**2019**:5364730. DOI: 10.1155/2019/5364730

[69] Kijmanawat A, Panburana P, Reutrakul S, Tangshewinsirikul C. Effects of probiotic supplements on insulin resistance in gestational diabetes mellitus: A double-blind randomized controlled trial. Journal of Diabetes Investigation. 2019;**10**(1):163-170. DOI: 10.1111/jdi.12863

Section 3

Consequences of Gestational Diabetes Mellitus

Chapter 7

GDM-Induced Vascular Injury and Its Relationship with Fetal Metabolic Impairment

Cristian Espinoza

Abstract

Cardiovascular diseases are a significant health problem worldwide. To date, there is a lack of awareness that perinatal factors can predispose to CVD before birth. Gestational diabetes mellitus is an increasingly prevalent disease associated with poor fetal outcomes and CVD in the offspring. Evidence from the last decades suggests that GDM causes endothelial dysfunction and impairs nutrient transfer across the placenta to the fetus. These pathological features are associated with altered vascular and trophoblastic homeostasis in the placenta, predisposing the offspring to vascular injury, altered metabolic condition, and future CVD. This chapter focuses its discussion on the to-date understanding of GDM fetoplacental vascular and nutrient transfer impairment that causes, along with the latest advances, limitations, and questions that remain unresolved in this field.

Keywords: gestational diabetes mellitus, cardiovascular diseases, pregnancy, hyperglycemia, endothelial cells

1. Introduction

Almost one of every three adults worldwide dies because of cardiovascular diseases (CVD), making them the most prevalent cause of morbidity and mortality [1]. Several factors increase the risk of suffering a CVD. They can divide into two groups: modifiable and non-modifiable [2]. The former are those factors that can be controlled and modified by behavior, such as physical activity and diet, while the latter ones cannot be changed, like age and genetics. Environmental factors include air pollution and exposure to heavy metals, such as arsenic or lead, and the WHO recognizes them as important CVD risk factors. They could be considered "modifiable"; however, considering that most of the population affected by environmental pollution live in medium to low-income countries, their modification might be complex. An excellent review on this topic was published elsewhere [3]. The apparition of pathological conditions during pregnancy such as pre-eclampsia [4], maternal supraphysiological hypercholesterolemia (MSPH) [5], or gestational diabetes mellitus (GDM) [6] alters the fetal environment and is associated with an increase an increased risk of CVD in the offspring. They might be considered "between" modifiable and non-modifiable: In the gestational state, controlling the disease might prevent the fetal vascular impairment; however, after birth, there is a lack of evidence regarding treatments for improving their outcome and might be considered a non-modifiable factor. Most of the published research focuses on the repercussions of maternal health after suffering pregnancy disease [7, 8]. Still, their effects on the cardiovascular health of the fetus have been less described.

Over the last decades, the evidence associating pregnancy diseases and fetal outcomes has grown. Regarding MSPH, the apparition of fatty streaks on tunica intima of large arteries at fetal stages [9], probably related to alterations in nutrient transfer through the placenta [10], increases the risk of future cardiovascular events. Sadly, this condition is frequently underdiagnosed [11], and for a solid understanding of its prognosis more studies are needed. Preeclampsia is a relatively common complication of pregnancy [12]. It is associated with a slight but sustained increase in diastolic and systolic pressure on the offspring that seems to maintain for life [13, 14]. Preeclampsia also is related to Intrauterine Growth Restriction [15], which, in turn, is associated with an impaired vascular and metabolic condition [16], predisposing the offspring to worst cardiovascular outcomes. Finally, GDM is a more common disease with global prevalence between 6 and 7% (Europe and United States) and 9 and 13% (South and Central America, Asia, Africa) [17]. The prevalence over the last decades has been increasing in most countries [18–21]; this might relate to the increase in maternal body mass index and the age of a pregnancy [18]. In terms of fetal cardiovascular impairment, a recent meta-analysis found that the offspring whose gestation was affected by GDM present higher basal glucose and systolic pressure [6]. In another large study, GDM pregnancies increased the prevalence of early-onset CVD by almost 30% in the offspring [22]. This worldwide statistical information urges researchers and clinicians to study the repercussions of GDM-complicated pregnancies further. Even more, an association between GDM and preeclampsia has been recently described [23, 24]. This relation can be explained at a systemic level by the increase in the age at which women become pregnant and the augment in body mass index told before; besides, both are related to damage on endothelial cells (EC), impairing vascular homeostasis [23]. Finally, between GDM and MSPH, a relation was recently suggested [25, 26], where EC in the placental vasculature and trophoblasts might have a crucial role; however, there is a considerable lack of evidence in this regard. At this point seems fair to suggest that EC is essential for the pathological development of the three conditions mentioned above. We will explore the GDM-induced vascular and trophoblastic injury and how it can probably impair fetal vascular health in the following pages.

1.1 Gestational diabetes mellitus pathophysiology

GDM is the apparition of spontaneous hyperglycemia in pregnancy without the previous diagnosis of a condition whose main feature is insulin resistance (IR) [27]. This definition is consistent with the evidence that GDM pathophysiology differs from pregnancies of women with prior diabetes in multiple aspects [28] as discussed later.

During a healthy pregnancy, the peripheral insulin sensitivity variates: In the early gestation increases to promote the fill up the glycogen and adipose stores [29], later it declines [30], increasing maternal systemic and placental glycemia. This reduction of insulin sensitivity (i.e., IR) occurs due to the pregnancy variation of systemic and placental hormones (for example, leptin, cortisol, estrogen, progesterone) [31] and is matched with a 2-fold increase in insulin secretion from pancreatic β-cells [32]. Late gestational hyperglycemia favors the transport of glucose to the fetus; however, it depletes the glycogen reservoirs and induces the use of fatty acids as fuel [33]. In GDM, maternal insulin sensitivity almost halves [34], implying two consequences: less accumulation of glycogen in both muscle and liver in the early pregnancy and faster use of them during late pregnancy. Furthermore, once the glycogen stores deplete, the use of fatty acids to obtain energy is more pronounced than in physiological pregnancy, leading to hypertriglyceridemia (HTG) (**Figure 1**).

Nonetheless, the reader is invited to reflect that a broad spectrum of clinical conditions related to the variable peripheral state of IR can exist [35, 36]. Finally, HTG and hyperglycemia alter placental vasculature [37] and fetal metabolic homeostasis [22, 38]. These features will be the focus of the following sections.

1.2 Gestational diabetes mellitus diagnose

Even when most of the pathophysiological features are known, reaching a diagnostic criterion for GDM has been troublesome. Huhn et al. [39] recently published a review of this topic. To date, one of the most widely accepted definitions is from the International Association of Diabetes and Pregnancy Study Group (IADPSG) [40]. The American Diabetes Association (ADA) agreed with IADPSG; however, first, they suggested a more flexible criterion than IADPS [41]. **Table 1** summarizes both.

The main difference between IADPS and ADA criteria is that the former considers that only one of the mentioned values needs to be altered to diagnose GDM. At the same time, ADA suggests that at least two of them must be present to diagnose GDM [41]. This slight discrepancy seems to be clinically significant: IADPS diagnostic of GDM increases two-fold [42] or three-fold [43] compared to

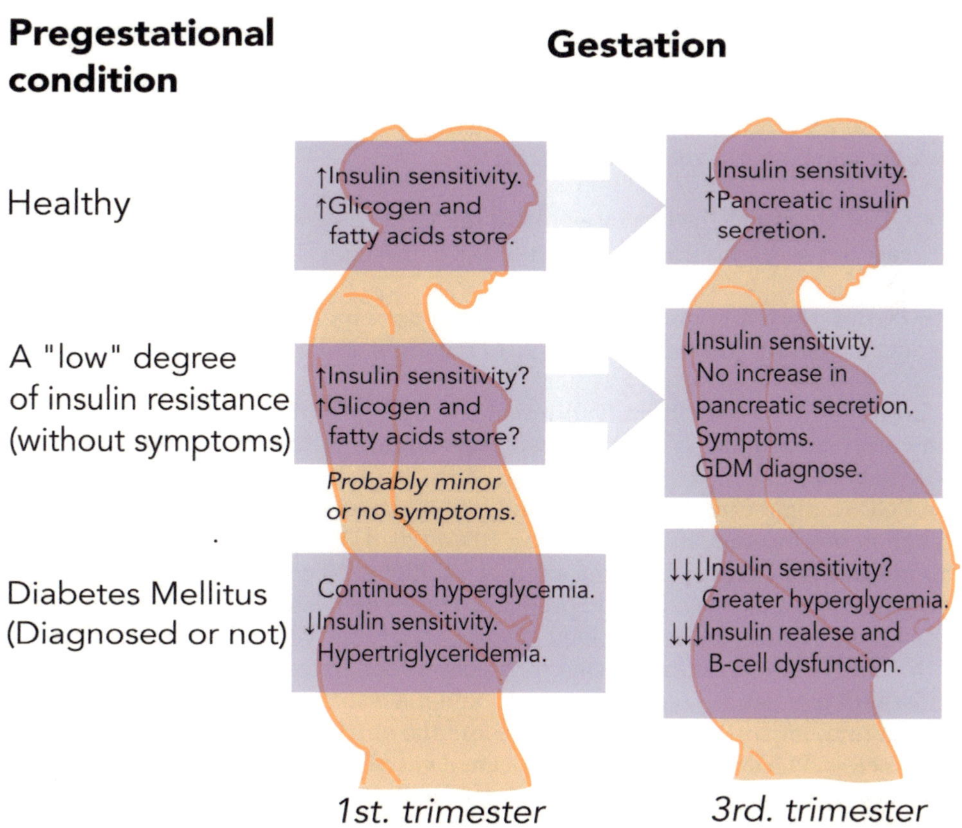

Figure 1.
Metabolic differences between first and third trimester in healthy pregnancies, with a low degree of IR and previously diagnosed Diabetes mellitus. Previous low degree of insulin resistance increases the risk of developing GDM in the third trimester; however, since it courses without significant symptoms, previous IR repercussions are not usually assessed. PGDM alters the placenta's formation in the first trimester, leading to more significant complications on the mother and the fetus in the third trimester.

Test	IADPSG	ADA
Fasting glucose	≥92 mg/dL	≥95 mg/dL
1-h glycemia after OGTT*	≥180 mg/dL	≥180 mg/dL
2-h glycemia after OGTT*	≥153 mg/dL	≥155 mg/dL

**OGTT: oral glucose tolerance test after a charge of 75 g of oral glucose.*
• Both entities consider that this evaluation must be performed between 24 and 28 weeks of gestation.
• The first sample must be taken after 8 h of fasting.

Table 1.
Diagnostic values for GDM.

ADA; moreover, using the IADPS criteria for diagnosis and treatment improves the adverse fetal outcomes of GDM [42, 43]. In this regard, ADA recent guidelines validated and included the IADPS criteria for GDM diagnosis [44].

1.3 Pregestational diabetes mellitus (PGDM)

Women's pregestational condition has historically complexed the study of GDM. GDM tends to appear in women with a previous degree of IR, and insufficient insulin synthesis or release from the pancreas before gravidity [40]. However, for decades, GDM was described as "any degree of glucose intolerance with onset or first recognition during pregnancy" [42, 45], regardless of the prior existence of unrecognized IR. This definition implies a severe limitation. The test for GDM is usually performed between the second and third trimester; but the screening for metabolic perturbances on women at fertile age, before pregnancy, are not actively pursued or a worldwide practice. In this regard, at the time of the GDM diagnose, there are two potential scenarios (**Figure 1**):

- GDM "de novo": the increase of IR at the third trimester will trigger the disease, leading both mother and fetus to a trimester of hyperglycemia and HTG.

- PGDM: the entire pregnancy will occur under a higher IR state, only being detected (and treated) from the third trimester and onwards.

Both conditions are clinically different. For example, birth weight over 4 kg, known as macrosomia, is associated with several fetal metabolic complications [46]. GDM is a risk factor of macrosomia; however, it has been recently suggested that PGDM might cause more severe and frequent metabolic complications, including macrosomia, in the fetus than GDM [28, 47]. A possible explanation for this might rely on more prolonged exposure to higher IR consequences, such as hyperglycemia and HTG. HTG in pregnancy on its own is associated with macrosomia [48]; besides, increased blood glucose, the primary manifestation of both GDM and PGDM, is also associated with poorer fetal outcomes [6, 49]. Both cause oxidative stress [50, 51], cytokine release, and meta-inflammation [52] in the forming placenta, impairing its ultrastructure and the nutrient transport to the fetus. Nonetheless, PGDM will expose the placental vasculature since its early formation to HTG and hyperglycemia. In the next sections, we will extensively discuss this topic.

1.4 Gestational diabetes mellitus induced vascular injury

As stated before, hyperglycemia and HTG are characteristic features of GDM and cause vascular injury on the placenta. Same as what happens on type 2 diabetes mellitus, GDM altered glucose metabolism on placental vasculature increases the production of reactive oxygen species (ROS) leading to oxidative stress (OS) [53, 54]. OS, in turn, favors the activation of Nuclear Factor kappa Beta and other pro-inflammatory pathways [55]. In GDM, the placenta itself expresses inflammatory cytokines [56]. Inflammation and OS will further induce systemic and placental IR, reducing the entry of glucose to cells [32, 57], impairing glycogen synthesis at the muscle and liver, leading to hyperglycemia and HTG. This oxidative and inflammatory state will also induce endothelial dysfunction (ED) impairing the vascular response to tissular metabolic needs, altering nutrient transfer to the fetus, and increasing the expression of adhesion molecules. To understand better the pathophysiological features of GDM on placental blood vessels and how it impairs the fetal metabolic condition, it is necessary first to summarize the main characteristics of the human placenta.

1.4.1 Development of the placental vascular system

In this section, we will explore the main features of placental development. For an in-depth study on this topic, the reader is invited to review the recent publication done by Turco et al. [58]. In brief, after the fertilization, the zygote will course with successive divisions forming the blastocyst, which will, in turn, adhere to the endometrium and invade it. The most external epithelial layer of the blastocyst will produce various trophoblast cell types and generate the primary syncytium below the implanted embryo [59]. The outer trophoblasts cells will differentiate and fusion, creating the syncytiotrophoblasts [60], whereas the inner cells will differentiate in cytotrophoblast. The syncytiotrophoblasts invade the endometrium and give rise to lacunas, spaces filled with maternal blood that will enlarge, merge, and develop the trabecular system of the forming placenta. The structure formed by both cell types around the lacunae is the primary villi. Later, the fetal mesenchyme will penetrate the villous core forming a structure known as secondary villi. Finally, vascular capillaries will appear within the center of fetal mesenchyme, forming the tertiary villi after the third gestation week. In the following weeks, angiogenesis predominates, increasing capillary density in the villi by developing new branches from preexisting vessels. Thus, the surface area for nutrient and oxygen exchange between the mother and the fetus increase [61]. At this point, in terms of vascular development, the placenta has reached its maturity (**Figure 2**). It is important to note that there are other essential structures in placentogenesis; however, they are beyond the scope of this chapter.

1.4.2 Diabetes impact on placental vascular formation

Tertiary villi arise at half of the second trimester. The pathological difference between PGDM and GDM becomes essential at this stage: from the implantation, and onwards, PGDM will expose the trophoblastic layer to an insulin-resistant, hyperglycemic, and hypoxic environment. Exploring the detrimental effects of both conditions is complicated since it needs the interruption of the pregnancy in human studies. Nonetheless, recent data permitted insight into the alterations caused by GDM or PGDM on the early placenta.

Spiral arteries in the endometrium are invaded by trophoblasts and remodeled [62]. This remodeling turns them into a resistance vessel, favoring the fell of arterial pressure, increasing placental blood flow. This process occurs by a coordinated proliferation, differentiation, and invasion of the trophoblasts, further forming the placenta. Several growth factors, including insulin-like growth factor I (IGF-I), and II (IGF-II) among others, released from the same trophoblasts [63] and other

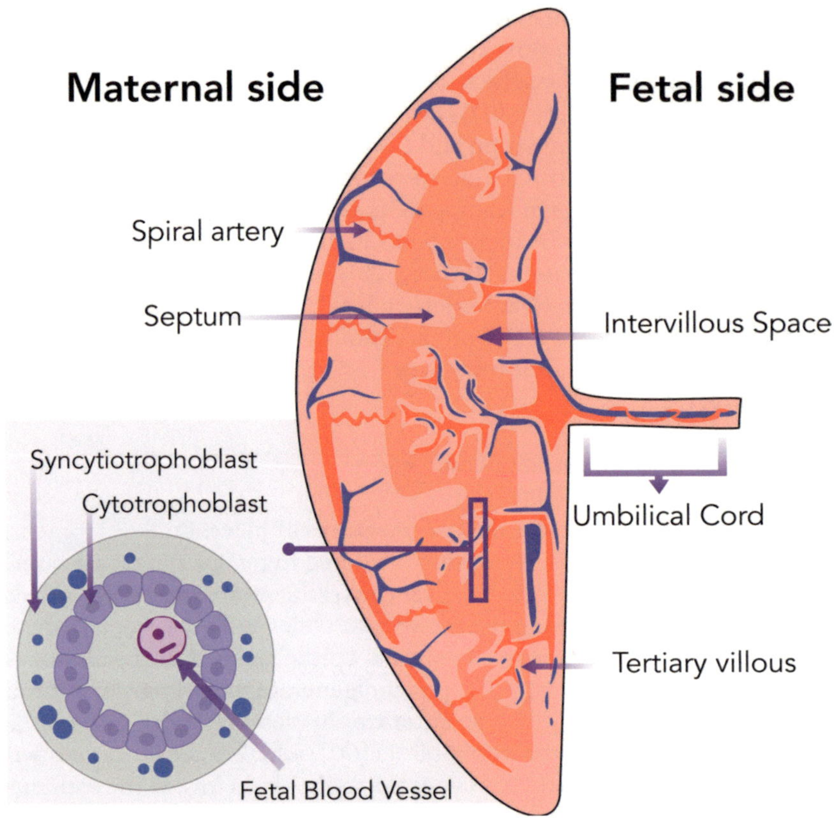

Figure 2.
The human term placenta. Maternal blood reaches the intervillous space (lacunae) through spiral arteries. Then, nutrients and oxygen cross the cytotrophoblasts from the microvillous membrane to the basal membrane and gets to the fetal blood vessels.

placental cell types, stimulate this process [64]. The placenta of GDM is heavier than healthy pregnancies, at least from the second trimester [65] and onwards [66]. This process is not fully understood; however, some findings have elucidated the role of growth factors. Placentas of IR pregnancies have an increased number of cytotrophoblasts, syncytiotrophoblasts, and EC due to a higher proliferation rate [64]. Consequently, placental vascularization in GDM is also enhanced by increased angiogenesis [67]. Differences in expression and secretion of growth factors from GDM trophoblasts themselves seem likely [68]. This increase in proliferation and angiogenesis has been shown in term placentas [68, 69]; yet, a recent study found that high IR is associated with a decrease in trophoblasts' proliferation and increased apoptosis on first-trimester placentas [70]. Another recent work suggested that hyperinsulinemia can also exert those detrimental effects [71]. Apoptosis is low in early healthy pregnancies placentas [72], progressively increasing until term [73]. On GDM, apoptosis analysis has led to conflicting results, showing a decrease [74] or an increase [75] in term placentas. Different technical approaches or the criteria used to diagnose GDM might explain these discrepancies; therefore, more detailed studies are needed. In summary, IR impairs the signaling of growth factors on vascular and trophoblast cells, diminishing the development and invasion respectively at the first trimester; however, as gestation progresses, more growth factors are secreted in a compensatory manner further increasing the size, weight, and the number of blood vessels in the placenta.

Among growth factors, IGF-I and IGF-II are potent stimulators of placental vascular growth, acting through their cognate receptor or insulin receptor. It is important to note that the insulin receptor has two isoforms: A and B. Isoform B presents a sequence of 12 amino acids in the α subunit that A does not have. This slight difference gives them different intracellular signaling and substrate affinity. Isoform A is associated with a mitogenic phenotype via mitogen-activated protein kinases (MAPK), while Isoform B induces metabolic modulation via protein kinase B (Akt). Moreover, IGF-II interaction with insulin receptor A induces cell growth and invasion, while insulin activity on the same isoform protects from apoptosis [76]. This differential action may explain the differences observed in the regulation of apoptosis and cell cycle described above. Exposure to increased insulin levels reduces the insulin receptor and IGF-I receptor's signaling via insulin response element I and downstream targets such as Akt [63]. At this point seems fair to hypothesize that IR impairs placental vascular development by altering the insulin and IGF-I receptor signaling, dysregulating proliferation, and apoptosis. This impairment might explain the high immaturity level of the villous observed in the GDM placenta [77]. Concordant with this hypothesis, human umbilical veins endothelial cells (HUVEC) increase MAPK signaling probably via isoform A of the insulin receptor in GDM [78]. Insulin exposure reestablishes the downstream signaling and membrane expression of both isoforms [78], making it an attractive therapeutic alternative; however, the effectiveness of insulin is highly dependent on the previous IR state. Indeed, obese women that develop GDM respond worse to insulin treatment than lean, diminishing the insulin receptor presence at the membrane and lesser downstream signaling [79, 80]. It is important to note that maternal obesity does not mean necessary IR; however, since most studies do not present evidence from the pregestational state, this suggestion seems fair to be made. More studies are needed taking this consideration since insulin does not seem to be always the better option. An excellent review on this matter has been published elsewhere [81].

Finally, disruption of insulin and IGF receptors signaling, observed in IR states, is related to insufficient trophoblasts invasion, pregnancy-associated hypertension, and increased pregnancy complications, including abortion [63]. In this regard, insulin signaling in the placenta seems crucial and will focus on in the next section.

1.4.3 Placental vasomotor alterations on GDM

The human placenta has no autonomic innervation, so vascular tone regulation is performed by the myogenic tone and humoral and metabolic factors. Humoral factors include norepinephrine [82], renin-angiotensin system (RAS), and vasopressin [83]. The three of them impair invasion of the trophoblast in spiral arteries and alter placental vascular homeostasis. This phenomenon has been studied in pre-eclampsia; however, in GDM, there is a lack of evidence pointing to its potential pathological role. Strikingly, GDM increases the risk of pre-eclampsia from the first trimester and onwards [84]. Indeed, GDM curses with some of the same pre-eclampsia's placental vascular complications (i.e., placental hypoxia and ED) [85]. In particular, maternal vasopressin does not seem to affect fetal blood flow [86], same as norepinephrine [87]. Nonetheless, the latter is related to a reduction in fetal oxygen delivery. This is likely to happen in pregnancies of women with prior diabetes [88] and GDM [89]: both conditions increase catecholamines plasmatic concentration in part because of hyperglycemia [90]. Moreover, norepinephrine augments IR [91, 92], and epinephrine diminishes insulin secretion from the pancreas [93]. In summary, upregulation of catecholamines in GDM negatively impacts placental vessel homeostasis; however, further studies are needed to explore this issue.

Several studies have highlighted the physiological role of the RAS system in placental development and function. A review in this regard has been recently published elsewhere [94]. In brief, the placenta presents all the components of RAS [95]. After implantation, tissular hypoxia induces syncytiotrophoblast formation, the remodeling of the spiral arteries, and angiogenesis. Angiotensin II receptor 1 (AT1R) expression is increased by hypoxia in trophoblasts and spiral arteries, augmenting the expression of angiogenic factors [96]. In healthy pregnancies, AT1R is highly expressed in the trophoblasts in the first and second trimester, declining its levels on the third [97]. However, if hypoxia persists, the expression of AT1R remains high until the end of the pregnancy [98]. As mentioned above, GDM incurs placental hypoxia, which might increase AT1R expression in trophoblasts [99], vascularity in the placenta and placental weight. AT1R expression due to GDM also increases in other vascular beds in rodent models, increasing vascular resistance and systemic arterial pressure [99]. Further, GDM increases the plasma concentration of angiotensin II (AGII), and permanent exposure to AGII induces vasoconstriction, diminishing placental blood flow and fetal oxygen delivery [100]. Also, IR in GDM may cause hyperinsulinemia, which in turn enhances the AT1R [101] and AGII [102] expression. In this regard, the relation between RAS and GDM seems to be even more complex. Higher plasma levels of soluble renin/prorenin receptor in the early pregnancy relate to an increased risk of developing GDM in late pregnancy [103]. This observation is in concordance with the fact that inhibitors of RAS, such as losartan, improve the vascular condition in human diabetes [104, 105] and rodent models of GDM [106]. Furthermore, GDM also increases the plasma concentration of aldosterone [107], an end product of RAS. Interestingly, hyperaldosteronism is associated with ED [108], which will be the subject of the following section. Nevertheless, to the best of my knowledge, this issue has not been assessed on fetoplacental vessels of GDM. Finally, increased AGII umbilical cord levels are associated with increased IR in GDM offspring [109]. Lesser perfusion of the β-cells can explain this due to vasoconstriction and a reduction of insulin sensitivity [110]. Indeed, blockade of RAS ameliorates IR [111]. Both processes converge in EC, where AGII increases ROS production, favoring oxidative stress (OS) [112]. In turn, GDM placenta incurs in OS [54], which impairs insulin signaling in multiple points and induces an inflammatory response mediated by Nuclear Factor kappa B, JNK, and p38 MAPK [113]. On the other hand, AT1R stimulation increases the apoptosis in villous explants and trophoblasts, which associates with pre-eclampsia [114], an event that might also happen in GDM; however, further studies are needed to explore this intricate process.

1.4.4 Endothelial dysfunction on GDM

ED is characterized by imbalanced vasodilation and vasoconstriction, elevated ROS, inflammation, and a deficit of nitric oxide (NO) bioavailability [115, 116]. All these phenomena occur in the GDM placenta, leading to an increased vascular tone and reduced perfusion.

Arachidonic acid is the precursor of thromboxane A2 (TXA2), a vasoconstrictor, and prostacyclin, a vasodilator. The synthesis of both can occur in EC. TXA2 acts through the TXA2 receptor (TR), present in the human umbilical vein. Besides, non-enzymatic oxidation of arachidonic acid produces isoprostanes [117], which can also interact with TR and induce constriction. GDM placentas show an increased synthesis of isoprostanes [54], probably due to the increased production of ROS. In GDM [118] and preeclampsia [119] the prostacyclin/TXA2 ratio is lower in the placenta. Interestingly, OS in trophoblasts increases the concentration of TXA2 but not prostacyclin, pointing to ROS as the responsible for this mechanism that increases the vascular tone. Endothelium-derived hyperpolarization (EDH) is mostly unexplored in placental vessels, yet it may play a role in GDM placental vascular impairment. EDH exerts vasodilation via stimulation of the Ca^{2+}-activated K^{+} channels, which hyperpolarize vascular smooth muscle cells (VSMC) [120]. It is hard to guess if GDM alters this mechanism. Preeclamptic pregnancies show a lesser EDH effect [121]; however, type 2 diabetes mellitus increases the EDH effect [122]. Further studies are needed to elucidate if EDH impairs or compensates ED in GDM.

Nitric oxide (NO) is probably the most characterized endothelium-derived vasodilator agent. Indeed, some consider that NO is the most potent vasodilator in the human placenta [123]. Due to its biological relevance, it is not surprising that its bioavailability is highly regulated. For instance, NO depends on the cellular intake of L-Arginine and the activity of the nitric oxide synthases. In EC, endothelial nitric oxide synthase (eNOS) is the primary source of NO, and cytosolic calcium, protein kinase A, and AKT favor the activity of this enzyme [124]. Insulin stimulates eNOS via AKT; besides, diabetes impairs this stimulation reducing eNOS activity, while reduction of NO induces IR, forming a vicious cycle [125]. On the other hand, NO acts on the VSMC, causing dilation via guanylyl-cyclase; however, it favors apoptosis [126] and inhibits proliferation [127] of the same cell type. VSMC apoptosis reduces the capability of resistance vessels to contract; in contrast, AGII favors proliferation via ROS activation of p38 MAPK [128]. Interestingly, a recent publication observed that GDM increases the insulin receptor isoform A and IGF 1R [129]. This gives consistency to the observations stated before: GDM enhances RAS and insulin receptor isoform A signaling in the placenta, both favoring the proliferation of VSMC; however, even when the machinery to produce NO upregulates in GDM [130], a reduction in its bioavailability is observed probably due to depletion by oxidative stress [131]. In turn, NO reduction inhibits apoptosis and further favors proliferation of VSMC, which will increase vascular tone, reduce perfusion, increasing hypoxia, and stimulate angiogenesis and even more OS. Nonetheless, even when consistent, this idea (**Figure 3**) needs further experimental support.

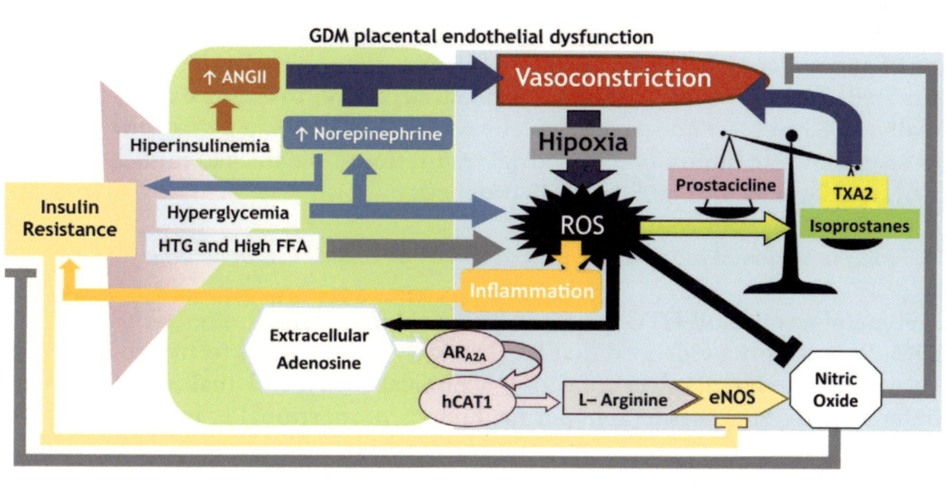

Figure 3.
Mechanisms of GDM-induced endothelial dysfunction in the human placenta. Insulin resistance, hyperinsulinemia, hyperglycemia, hypertriglyceridemia (HTG), and high plasma concentration of free fatty acids (FFA) characterize GDM. These alterations induce vasoconstriction, hypoxia, and reactive oxygen species (ROS) production. ROS, in turn, will increase thromboxane A2 (TxA2) and isoprostanes in endothelial cells, further favoring vasoconstriction. ROS also upregulates the adenosine signaling, and the adenosine/L-Arginine/nitric oxide axis will be upregulated; however, insulin resistance diminishes endothelial nitric oxide synthase (eNOS) phosphorylation and nitric oxide (NO) production. Also, ROS will interact with NO and produce peroxynitrite, reducing NO bioavailability.

L-Arginine also determines the synthesis of NO by eNOS. L-Arginine is transformed in L-citrulline for NO production by eNOS [123]; so, NO production is dependent on intracellular L-Arginine content. Cationic amino acid transporter 1 (hCAT-1) is the main responsible for the entry of L-Arginine to the cell in the human [132]. Interestingly, insulin, OS and the activation of adenosine receptor A 2A (AR_{A2A}) induce hCAT-1 expression [133]. In this regard, even when in GDM impairs insulin signaling, OS and the activation of AR_{A2A} will favor the expression of hCAT-1 and secure the L-Arginine entry. OS can also induce the activation of adenosine receptor [134]. However, the insulin effect over hCAT-1 expression and activity has been described as requiring functional AR_{A2A} in HUVEC [135]. GDM hinders adenosine transport to the cell, increasing its extracellular concentration [136, 137]. Extracellular adenosine will activate AR_{A2A}, which will induce vasodilation [133]. Interestingly, adenosine can also interact with adenosine receptor A 2B (AR_{A2B}), which is expressed in microvascular EC and induces angiogenesis [138]. The high adenosine concentration facilitates the AR_{A2B} activation and may relate to the increased vascularization and weight observed in GDM placentas. A recent work has shown that adenosine induces fetal vessels constriction; however, GDM impairs its vasoconstrictor effect [139]. Going back to the above, even when the whole adenosine/L-Arginine/NO axis raises in GDM, the lesser bioavailability of NO impedes its biological effect. Likewise, NO deficit might explain why GDM reduces the insulin vasodilatory effect [131]. In this regard, endothelial dysfunction by GDM not only affects vasodilation but vasoconstriction as well, hindering the capability of the endothelium to regulate the vascular tone.

Finally, it is crucial to note that hypoxia [140] and hyperglycemia [141] induce OS. Interestingly, hyperglycemia on its own can induce hypoxia [142]. Mitochondrial impairment is probably the most important source of ROS in GDM; an excellent review has been made elsewhere [143]. Further, a recent work described mitochondrial dysfunction in cytotrophoblast and syncytiotrophoblast from GDM pregnancies. The latter seems to be more comprised in terms of ATP generation and increases the expression of antioxidants [144]. Nonetheless, this impairment is more profound when higher grades of IR are present [113] and the pregestational condition is highly relevant [143]. Insulin can increase the production of antioxidants; however, in GDM placentas, the expression of antioxidants is increased constantly [145], making them less responsive to future oxidants insults. Finally, ROS can react non-enzymatically with NO, producing peroxynitrite, which has been shown to inhibit mitochondrial respiration and damaged mitochondria [146], making a vicious cycle for ROS production.

1.4.5 Placental altered nutrient transfer on GDM and fetal metabolic injury

Hyperglycemia and HTG are the most common metabolic alterations in GDM. Recent work evidenced that HTG in early pregnancy is related to IR, β-cell dysfunction, and hyperglycemia [147]. Umbilical cord blood analysis has demonstrated that GDM causes fetal hyperinsulinemia proportional to maternal IR [148]. Triglyceridemia remains unaltered, but LDL concentrations increase and HDL diminishes in cord blood of GDM deliveries and directly associates with macrosomia [149]. Intriguingly, triglyceridemia remains unaltered since maternal HTG is better related to macrosomia than hyperglycemia itself [150–152]. In this regard, the relationship observed between HTG and macrosomia in GDM might have two possible causes: an increase in the fetal delivery of free fatty acids (FFA) posterior to the action of lipases or the impairment of placental homeostasis due to ED. The first hypothesis does not seem likely: even when GDM curses with high FFA maternal plasma concentration [153], cord blood FFA content remains unaltered in GDM deliveries [154]. In this regard, the second hypothesis seems more plausible. HTG is related to ED; however, a mechanistic explanation is lacking to date. A recent review was made about this topic elsewhere [155]. A probable explanation for ED lies in macrophage activation by triglyceride-rich lipoproteins like Very-Low-Density Lipoprotein (VLDL) [156]. VLDL also induces ROS production and expression of inflammation mediators such as Tumoral Necrosis Factor α (TNF-α) in EC [157]. Interestingly, TNF-α favors IR and hyperinsulinemia in GDM [32], hindering insulin-mediated vasodilation. Also, the oxidative environment induced by triglycerides may favor the NO consumption, establishing the ED. Nonetheless, further studies are needed to address this issue in GDM placentas.

Finally, glucose transport in the placenta is regulated by maternal glycemia and by the expression and activity of glucose transporters (GLUT). For transportation from the mother to the fetus, glucose must go through the microvillous membrane (MVM), at the maternal side, to the basal membrane (BM) on the fetal side [158]. At least 6 GLUT transporters have been identified in the placenta: GLUT1, GLUT3, GLUT4, GLUT8, GLUT9, and GLUT12. Nonetheless, the most abundant isoforms in the placenta are GLUT1 and GLUT4. GLUT1 levels increase in syncytiotrophoblasts along with the pregnancy progression [159]. GLUT1 expresses in the MVM 3-fold than in the BM. Thus, crossing the BM is the rate-limiting step for glucose transport to fetal circulation [160]. Indeed, increased content of GLUT1 is correlated proportionally with fetal weight and macrosomia [161]. GLUT4 expression, contrarily to what was thought before [159], increases during gestation in the MVM, but only in healthy lean women [162]. In GDM, interestingly, insulin lowers mRNA of GLUT4; besides, various authors found increased GLUT1 expression [79, 163, 164]. Even more, GLUT1 upregulation is more profound in PGDM [164]. In this regard, it seems fair to suggest that GLUT 1 in the BM is critical for GDM pregnancy complications due to increased glucose transport [165]. Hyperglycemia should limit GLUT1 expression in trophoblasts and favor its movement from the membrane to the cytoplasm [166, 167]; however, in GDM, this does not seem to happen. A mechanistic study is necessary to address this issue. Finally, an increased transfer of maternal insulin to the fetus could explain hyperinsulinemia observed in the fetal cord of GDM deliveries. Nonetheless, near 1% maternal insulin crosses the placenta [168]. This could hardly cause an increase in fetal insulinemia; however, it may contribute. In this regard, the Modified Pedersen hypothesis offers a better explanation: Maternal hyperglycemia passes through the placenta to the fetus; then, from the second trimester and onwards, the fetal pancreas responds to hyperglycemia with hyperinsulinemia, further favoring glucose disposition in fat stores and the anabolic effects of insulin, resulting in macrosomia [169]. This could also explain the vascular alterations observed in the GDM offspring; however, further research for addressing this issue is needed.

2. Conclusion

GDM is a complex condition that affects both fetus and mother. Its impact on the offspring includes vascular and metabolic impairment before birth, predisposing them to early CVD. The real prevalence of GDM worldwide is unknown and might go beyond our expectations since it is mostly underdiagnosed. Moreover, the differential impact of previously diagnosed diabetes in pregnancy has begun to elucidate in the last few decades. On the other hand, the reader is invited to reflect that the pathological IR state in pregnancy is not a "black-or-white" matter but a continuous spectrum of possible conditions and fetal outcomes that needs to be assessed in every pregnancy individually. Including the assessment of HbA1c and lipid profile test in the first trimester, evaluation might improve the diagnosis of PGDM and foresee the future GDM development.

Previous IR state and PGDM hinder syncytiotrophoblast invasion in maternal vessels and the placenta formation; however, there is still much to research and learn from this subject. After development, GDM will continuously expose the placenta to a hypoxic environment that will impair vascular function due to increased OS and inflammation. HTG, hyperglycemia, and increased FFA will favor this pro-oxidant environment, causing ED. The regulation of the vascular tone by EC will impair favoring vasoconstriction and further tissular hypoxia. The nutrient transfer to the fetus will alter on this condition, exposing it constantly to hyperglycemia. Persistent hyperglycemia will damage its blood vessels and force its β-cells to secrete insulin extensively, causing metabolic and vascular impairment that will predispose it to CVD before its birth.

Acknowledgements

Especial thanks to Tamara Jiménez Iturrieta for the illustrations.
The author declares that no funding was received for this publication.

Conflict of interest

The authors declare no conflict of interest.

Nomenclature

ADA	American Diabetes Association
AGII	angiotensin II
AT1R	angiotensin II receptor 1
AR_{A2A}	adenosine receptor A 2A
AR_{A2B}	adenosine receptor A 2B
BM	basal membrane
CVD	cardiovascular diseases
EC	endothelial cells
ED	endothelial dysfunction
eNOS	endothelial nitric oxide synthase
EDH	endothelium-derived hyperpolarization
FFA	free fatty acids
GDM	gestational diabetes mellitus
HTG	hypertriglyceridemia
hCAT-1	human cationic amino acid transporter 1
HUVEC	human umbilical veins endothelial cells
IGF-I	insulin-like growth factor I
IGF-II	insulin-like growth factor II
IR	insulin resistance
IADPSG	International Association of Diabetes and Pregnancy Study Group
MSPH	maternal supraphysiological hypercholesterolemia
MVM	microvillous membrane
MAPK	mitogen-activated protein kinases
NO	nitric oxide
OS	oxidative stress

DOI: http://dx.doi.org/10.5772/intechopen.102626

PGDM	pregestational diabetes mellitus
Akt	protein kinase B
ROS	reactive oxygen species
RAS	renin-angiotensin system
TXA2	thromboxane A2
TR	thromboxane A2 receptor
TNF-α	tumoral necrosis factor α
VSMC	vascular smooth muscle cells

Author details

Cristian Espinoza[1,2]

1 Faculty of Biological Sciences, Pontifical Catholic University of Chile, Santiago, Chile

2 Faculty of Medicine, School of Nursing, Finis Terrae University, Providencia, Chile

*Address all correspondence to: espinoza.calvo.cristian@gmail.com

References

[1] McAloon CJ, Boylan LM, Hamborg T, Stallard N, Osman F, Lim PB, et al. The changing face of cardiovascular disease 2000-2012: An analysis of the world health organisation global health estimates data. International Journal of Cardiology. 2016;**224**:256-264

[2] National Heart, Lung and blood I. "What Are the Risk Factors for Heart Disease?" [Internet]. 2017. Available from: https://www.nhlbi.nih.gov/health-topics/education-and-awareness/heart-truth

[3] Cosselman KE, Navas-acien A, Kaufman JD. Environmental factors in cardiovascular disease. Nature Reviews. Cardiology. 2015;**12**(November): 627-642

[4] Hakim J, Senterman MK, Hakim AM. Preeclampsia is a biomarker for vascular disease in both mother and child: The need for a medical alert system. Kumar P, editor. International Journal of Pediatrics. 2013;**2013**:953150. DOI: 10.1155/2013/953150

[5] Napoli C, Glass CK, Witztum JL, Deutsch R, D'Armiento FP, Palinski W. Influence of maternal hypercholesterolaemia during pregnancy on progression of early atherosclerotic lesions in childhood: Fate of early lesions in children (FELIC) study. Lancet. 1999;**354**:1234-1241

[6] Pathirana MM, Lassi ZS, Roberts CT, Andraweera PH. Cardiovascular risk factors in offspring exposed to gestational diabetes mellitus in utero: Systematic review and meta-analysis. Journal of Developmental Origins of Health and Disease. 2019;**11**(October): 599-616

[7] Benschop L, Duvekot JJ, Van Lennep JER. Future risk of cardiovascular disease risk factors and events in women after a hypertensive disorder of pregnancy. Heart (British Cardiac Society). 2019;**76**:1273-1278

[8] Kramer CK, Campbell S, Retnakaran R. Gestational diabetes and the risk of cardiovascular disease in women: A systematic review and meta-analysis. Diabetologia. 2019;**62**(6):905-914

[9] Napoli C, D'Armiento FP, Mancini FP, Postiglione A, Witztum JL, Palumbo G, et al. Fatty streak formation occurs in human fetal aortas and is greatly enhanced by maternal hypercholesterolemia. Intimal accumulation of low density lipoprotein and its oxidation precede monocyte recruitment into early atherosclerotic lesions. The Journal of Clinical Investigation. 1997;**100**(11):2680-2690

[10] Cantin C, Fuenzalida B, Leiva A. Maternal hypercholesterolemia during pregnancy: Potential modulation of cholesterol transport through the human placenta and lipoprotein profile in maternal and neonatal circulation. Placenta. 2020;**94**(December):26-33

[11] Leiva A, Salsoso R, Sáez T, Sanhueza C, Pardo F, Sobrevia L. Cross-sectional and longitudinal lipid determination studies in pregnant women reveal an association between increased maternal LDL cholesterol concentrations and reduced human umbilical vein relaxation. Placenta. 2015;**36**(8):895-902

[12] Yang Y, Le Ray I, Zhu J, Zhang J, Hua J, Reilly M. Preeclampsia prevalence, risk factors, and pregnancy outcomes in Sweden and China. JAMA Network Open. 2021;**4**(5):e218401-e218401. DOI: 10.1001/jamanetwork open.2021.8401

[13] Mamun AA, Kinarivala MK, O'Callaghan M, Williams G, Najman J, Callaway L. Does hypertensive disorder

of pregnancy predict offspring blood pressure at 21 years? Evidence from a birth cohort study. Journal of Human Hypertension [Internet]. 2012;**26**(5): 288-294. DOI: 10.1038/jhh.2011.35

[14] Davis EF, Lazdam M, Lewandowski AJ, Worton SA, Kelly B, Kenworthy Y, et al. Cardiovascular risk factors in children and young adults born to preeclamptic pregnancies: A systematic review. Pediatrics. 2012;**129**(6):e1552-e1561

[15] Odegård RA, Vatten LJ, Nilsen ST, Salvesen KA, Austgulen R. Preeclampsia and fetal growth. Obstetrics and Gynecology. 2000;**96**(6):950-955

[16] Menendez-Castro C, Rascher W, Hartner A. Intrauterine growth restriction - impact on cardiovascular diseases later in life. Molecular and Cellular Pediatrics. 2018;**5**(1):4. Available from: https://pubmed.ncbi.nlm.nih.gov/29560535

[17] Zhu Y, Zhang C. Prevalence of gestational diabetes and risk of progression to type 2 Diabetes: A global perspective. Current Diabetes Reports. 2016;**16**(1):7. Available from: https://pubmed.ncbi.nlm.nih.gov/26742932

[18] Lavery JA, Friedman AM, Keyes KM, Wright JD, Ananth CV. Gestational diabetes in the United States: Temporal changes in prevalence rates between 1979 and 2010. BJOG: An International Journal of Obstetrics & Gynaecology. 2017;**124**(5):804-813. DOI: 10.1111/1471-0528.14236

[19] Leng J, Shao P, Zhang C, Tian H, Zhang F, Zhang S, et al. Prevalence of gestational diabetes mellitus and its risk factors in Chinese pregnant women: A prospective population-based study in Tianjin, China. PLoS One. 2015;**10**(3): e0121029

[20] Ferrara A. Increasing prevalence of gestational diabetes mellitus. Diabetes Care [Internet]. 2007;**30**(Supplement 2): S141-S146. Available from: http://care.diabetesjournals.org/content/30/Supplement_2/S141.abstract

[21] Collier A, Abraham EC, Armstrong J, Godwin J, Monteath K, Lindsay R. Reported prevalence of gestational diabetes in Scotland: The relationship with obesity, age, socioeconomic status, smoking and macrosomia, and how many are we missing? Journal of Diabetes Investigation. 2017;**8**(2):161-167

[22] Yu Y, Arah OA, Liew Z, Cnattingius S, Olsen J, Sørensen HT, et al. Maternal diabetes during pregnancy and early onset of cardiovascular disease in offspring: Population based cohort study with 40 years of follow-up. BMJ. 2019;**367**:1-4

[23] Lee J, Ouh Y-T, Ahn KH, Hong SC, Oh M-J, Kim H-J, et al. Preeclampsia: A risk factor for gestational diabetes mellitus in subsequent pregnancy. PLoS One. 2017;**12**(5):e0178150-e0178150 Available from: https://pubmed.ncbi.nlm.nih.gov/28542483

[24] Plows JF, Stanley JL, Baker PN, Reynolds CM, Vickers MH. The pathophysiology of gestational diabetes mellitus. International Journal of Molecular Sciences. 2018;**19**(11):3342. Available from: https://pubmed.ncbi.nlm.nih.gov/30373146

[25] Contreras-Duarte S, Carvajal L, Fuenzalida B, Cantin C, Sobrevia L, Leiva A. Maternal dyslipidaemia in pregnancy with gestational diabetes mellitus: Possible impact on Foetoplacental vascular function and lipoproteins in the neonatal circulation. Current Vascular Pharmacology. 2017;**17**(1):52-71

[26] Espinoza C, Fuenzalida B, Leiva A. Increased fetal cardiovascular disease risk: Potential synergy between gestational diabetes mellitus and

maternal hypercholesterolemia. Current Vascular Pharmacology. 2021;**19**:1-23

[27] Classification and diagnosis of diabetes: Standards of medical care in diabetes-2018. Diabetes Care. 2018;**41**(Suppl. 1):S13-S27

[28] Yang G-R, Dye TD, Li D. Effects of pre-gestational diabetes mellitus and gestational diabetes mellitus on macrosomia and birth defects in upstate New York. Diabetes Research and Clinical Practice. 2019;**155**:107811

[29] Di Cianni G, Miccoli R, Volpe L, Lencioni C, Del Prato S. Intermediate metabolism in normal pregnancy and in gestational diabetes. Diabetes/Metabolism Research and Reviews. 2003;**19**(4):259-270

[30] Catalano PM. Trying to understand gestational diabetes. Diabetic Medicine [Internet]. 2014;**31**(3):273-281 Available from: https://pubmed.ncbi.nlm.nih.gov/24341419

[31] Catalano PM, Tyzbir ED, Roman NM, Amini SB, Sims EA. Longitudinal changes in insulin release and insulin resistance in nonobese pregnant women. American Journal of Obstetrics and Gynecology. 1991;**165** (6 Pt 1):1667-1672

[32] Barbour LA, McCurdy CE, Hernandez TL, Kirwan JP, Catalano PM, Friedman JE. Cellular mechanisms for insulin resistance in normal pregnancy and gestational diabetes. Diabetes Care. 2007;**30**(Suppl. 2):S112-S119

[33] Lain KY, Catalano PM. Metabolic changes in pregnancy. Clinical Obstetrics and Gynecology. 2007;**50**(4):938-948

[34] Friedman JE, Ishizuka T, Shao J, Huston L, Highman T, Catalano P. Impaired glucose transport and insulin receptor tyrosine phosphorylation in skeletal muscle from obese women with gestational diabetes. Diabetes. 1999;**48**(9):1807-1814

[35] Ryckman KK, Spracklen CN, Smith CJ, Robinson JG, Saftlas AF. Maternal lipid levels during pregnancy and gestational diabetes: A systematic review and meta-analysis. BJOG: An International Journal of Obstetrics and Gynaecology. 2015;**122**(5):643-651

[36] Wang J, Li Z, Lin L. Maternal lipid profiles in women with and without gestational diabetes mellitus. Medicine (Baltimore). 2019;**98**(16):e15320-e15320. Available from: https://pubmed.ncbi.nlm.nih.gov/31008986

[37] Leiva A, Pardo F, Ramírez MA, Farías M, Casanello P, Sobrevia L. Fetoplacental vascular endothelial dysfunction as an early phenomenon in the programming of human adult diseases in subjects born from gestational diabetes mellitus or obesity in pregnancy. Experimental Diabetes Research. 2011;**2011**:349286

[38] Marco LJ, McCloskey K, Vuillermin PJ, Burgner D, Said J, Ponsonby AL. Cardiovascular disease risk in the offspring of diabetic women: The impact of the intrauterine environment. Experimental Diabetes Research. 2012;**2012**:565160.

[39] Huhn EA, Rossi SW, Hoesli I, Göbl CS. Controversies in screening and diagnostic criteria for gestational diabetes in early and late pregnancy. Frontiers in Endocrinology (Lausanne). 2018;**9**:696. DOI: https://www.frontiersin.org/article/10.3389/fendo.2018.00696

[40] Buchanan TA, Xiang AH. Gestational diabetes mellitus. Journal of Clinical Investigation. 2005;**115**(3):485-491. Available from: https://pubmed.ncbi.nlm.nih.gov/15765129

[41] Association AD. Diagnosis and classification of diabetes mellitus. Diabetes Care. 2010;**33**(Supplement 1): S62-S69 Available from: https://care.diabetesjournals.org/content/33/Supplement_1/S62

[42] Shang M, Lin L. IADPSG criteria for diagnosing gestational diabetes mellitus and predicting adverse pregnancy outcomes. Journal of Perinatology. 2014;**34**(2):100-104

[43] Duran A, Sáenz S, Torrejón MJ, Bordiú E, del Valle L, Galindo M, et al. Introduction of IADPSG criteria for the screening and diagnosis of gestational diabetes mellitus results in improved pregnancy outcomes at a lower cost in a large Cohort of pregnant women: The St. Carlos gestational diabetes study. Diabetes Care. 2014;**37**(9):2442-2450. Available from: https://care.diabetesjournals.org/content/37/9/2442

[44] Association AD. 2. Classification and Diagnosis of Diabetes: Standards of Medical Care in Diabetes—2020. Diabetes Care. 2020;**43**(Supplement 1): S14-S31. Available from: https://care.diabetesjournals.org/content/43/Supplement_1/S14

[45] Yang X, Hsu-Hage B, Zhang H, Zhang C, Zhang Y, Zhang C. Women with impaired glucose tolerance during pregnancy have significantly poor pregnancy outcomes. Diabetes Care. 2002;**25**(9):1619-1624

[46] Araujo Júnior E, Peixoto AB, Zamarian ACP, Elito Júnior J, Tonni G. Macrosomia. Best Practice & Research. Clinical Obstetrics & Gynaecology. 2017;**38**:83-96

[47] Fong A, Serra A, Herrero T, Pan D, Ogunyemi D. Pre-gestational versus gestational diabetes: A population based study on clinical and demographic differences. Journal of Diabetes and its Complications. 2014;**28**(1):29-34

[48] Olmos PR, Rigotti A, Busso D, Berkowitz L, Santos JL, Borzone GR, et al. Maternal hypertriglyceridemia: A link between maternal overweight-obesity and macrosomia in gestational diabetes. Obesity (Silver Spring). 2014;**22**(10):2156-2163

[49] Schaefer UM, Songster G, Xiang A, Berkowitz K, Buchanan TA, Kjos SL. Congenital malformations in offspring of women with hyperglycemia first detected during pregnancy. American Journal of Obstetrics and Gynecology. 1997;**177**(5):1165-1171

[50] Ramírez-Emiliano J, Fajardo-Araujo ME, Zúñiga-Trujillo I, Pérez-Vázquez V, Sandoval-Salazar C, Órnelas-Vázquez JK. Mitochondrial content, oxidative, and nitrosative stress in human full-term placentas with gestational diabetes mellitus. Reproductive Biology and Endocrinology. 2017;**15**(1):26. DOI: 10.1186/s12958-017-0244-7

[51] Lappas M, Hiden U, Desoye G, Froehlich J, Hauguel-de Mouzon S, Jawerbaum A. The role of oxidative stress in the pathophysiology of gestational diabetes mellitus. Antioxidants & Redox Signaling. 2011;**15**(12):3061-3100

[52] Desoye G, Hauguel-De MS. The human placenta in gestational diabetes mellitus: The insulin and cytokine network. Diabetes Care. 2007;**30** (Suppl. 2):S120-S126

[53] Zhu C, Yang H, Geng Q, Ma Q, Long Y, Zhou C, et al. Association of oxidative stress biomarkers with gestational diabetes mellitus in pregnant women: A case-control study. PLoS One. 2015;**10**(4):e0126490

[54] Coughlan MT, Vervaart PP, Permezel M, Georgiou HM, Rice GE. Altered placental oxidative stress status in gestational diabetes mellitus. Placenta. 2004;**25**(1):78-84

[55] Lingappan K. NF-κB in oxidative stress. Current Opinion in Toxicology. 2018;**7**:81-86

[56] Radaelli T, Varastehpour A, Catalano P, Mouzon SH. Gestational diabetes induces placental genes for chronic stress and inflammatory pathways GDM alters expression profile of placental genes. Diabetes. 2003;**52**(September):2951-2958

[57] Pessler D, Rudich A, Bashan N. Oxidative stress impairs nuclear proteins binding to the insulin responsive element in the GLUT4 promoter. Diabetologia. 2001;**44**(12): 2156-2164

[58] Turco MY, Moffett A. Development of the human placenta. Development. 2019;**146**:22

[59] Knöfler M, Pollheimer J. Human placental trophoblast invasion and differentiation: A particular focus on Wnt signaling. Frontiers in Genetics. 2013;**4**:190. DOI: https://www.frontiersin.org/article/10.3389/fgene.2013.00190

[60] Gude NM, Roberts CT, Kalionis B, King RG. Growth and function of the normal human placenta. Thrombosis Research. 2004;**114**(5-6 SPEC. ISS): 397-407

[61] Cross JC, Nakano H, Natale DRC, Simmons DG, Watson ED. Branching morphogenesis during development of placental villi. Differentiation. 2006;**74**(7):393-401

[62] Pijnenborg R, Vercruysse L, Hanssens M. The uterine spiral arteries in human pregnancy: Facts and controversies. Placenta. 2006;**27**(9-10):939-958

[63] Mayama R, Izawa T, Sakai K, Suciu N, Iwashita M. Improvement of insulin sensitivity promotes extravillous trophoblast cell migration stimulated by insulin-like growth factor-I. Endocrine Journal. 2013;**60**(3):359-368

[64] Aires MB. Effects of maternal diabetes on trophoblast cells. World Journal of Diabetes. 2015;**6**(2):338

[65] Edu A, Teodorescu C, Dobjanschi CG, Socol ZZ, Teodorescu V, Matei A, et al. Placenta changes in pregnancy with gestational diabetes. Rom J Morphol Embryol = Revue Roumaine de Morphologie et d'Embryologie. 2016;**57**(2):507-512

[66] Taricco E, Radaelli T, Nobile de Santis MS, Cetin I. Foetal and placental weights in relation to maternal characteristics in gestational diabetes. Placenta. 2003;**24**(4):343-347

[67] Huynh J, Dawson D, Roberts D, Bentley-Lewis R. A systematic review of placental pathology in maternal diabetes mellitus. Placenta. 2015;**36**(2):101-114

[68] Loegl J, Nussbaumer E, Cvitic S, Huppertz B, Desoye G, Hiden U. GDM alters paracrine regulation of feto-placental angiogenesis via the trophoblast. Laboratory Investigation. 2017;**97**(4):409-418

[69] Unek G, Ozmen A, Mendilcioglu I, Simsek M, Korgun ET. Immunohistochemical distribution of cell cycle proteins p27, p57, cyclin D3, PCNA and Ki67 in normal and diabetic human placentas. Journal of Molecular Histology. 2014;**45**(1):21-34

[70] Bandres-Meriz J, Hoch D, Honeder S, Majali-Martinez A, Emilio H, Matthias S, et al. 93-OR: Low maternal Insulin sensitivity associates with DNA-related functions in human first-trimester trophoblast. Diabetes. 2020;**69**(Supplement 1). Available from: https://diabetes.diabetesjournals.org/content/69/Supplement_1/93-OR

[71] Vega M, Mauro M, Williams Z. Direct toxicity of insulin on the human

placenta and protection by metformin. Fertility and Sterility. 2019;**111**(3):489-496.e5

[72] Smith SC, Leung TN, To KF, Baker PN. Apoptosis is a rare event in first-trimester placental tissue. American Journal of Obstetrics and Gynecology. 2000;**183**(3):697-699

[73] Sharp AN, Heazell AEP, Crocker IP, Mor G. Placental apoptosis in health and disease. American Journal of Reproductive Immunology. 2010;**64**(3):159-169. Available from: https://pubmed.ncbi.nlm.nih.gov/20367628

[74] Magee TR, Ross MG, Wedekind L, Desai M, Kjos S, Belkacemi L. Gestational diabetes mellitus alters apoptotic and inflammatory gene expression of trophobasts from human term placenta. Journal of Diabetes and its Complications. 2014;**28**(4):448-459

[75] Sgarbosa F, Barbisan LF, Brasil MAM, Costa E, Calderon IMP, Gonçalves CR, et al. Changes in apoptosis and Bcl-2 expression in human hyperglycemic, term placental trophoblast. Diabetes Research and Clinical Practice. 2006;**73**(2):143-149

[76] Westermeier F, Sáez T, Arroyo P, Toledo F, Gutiérrez J, Sanhueza C, et al. Insulin receptor isoforms: An integrated view focused on gestational diabetes mellitus. Diabetes/Metabolism Research and Reviews. 2016;**32**(4):350-365

[77] Benirschke K, Kaufmann PB, R. Pathology of the Humanplacenta. 5th ed. New York: Springer; 2006

[78] Villalobos-Labra R, Silva L, Subiabre M, Araos J, Salsoso R, Fuenzalida B, et al. Akt/mTOR role in human Foetoplacental vascular Insulin resistance in diseases of pregnancy. Wadsack C, editor. Journal of Diabetes Research. 2017;**2017**:5947859. DOI: 10.1155/2017/5947859

[79] Colomiere M, Permezel M, Riley C, Desoye G, Lappas M. Defective insulin signaling in placenta from pregnancies complicated by gestational diabetes mellitus. European Journal of Endocrinology. 2009;**160**(4):567-578

[80] Pérez-Pérez A, Guadix P, Maymó J, Dueñas JL, Varone C, Fernández-Sánchez M, et al. Insulin and leptin signaling in placenta from gestational diabetic subjects. Hormone and metabolic research = Hormon- und Stoffwechselforschung = Hormones et métabolisme. 2016;**48**(1):62-69

[81] Subiabre M, Silva L, Toledo F, Paublo M, López MA, Boric MP, et al. Insulin therapy and its consequences for the mother, foetus, and newborn in gestational diabetes mellitus. Biochimica et Biophysica Acta (BBA)—Molecular Basis of Disease. 2018;**1864**(9):2949-2956. DOI: 10.1016/j.bbadis.2018.06.005

[82] Na K-H, Choi JH, Kim C-H, Kim K-S, Kim GJ. Altered expression of norepinephrine transporter and norepinephrine in human placenta cause pre-eclampsia through regulated trophoblast invasion. Clinical and Experimental Reproductive Medicine. 2013;**40**(1):12-22. Available from: https://pubmed.ncbi.nlm.nih.gov/23614111

[83] Opichka MA, Rappelt MW, Gutterman DD, Grobe JL, McIntosh JJ. Review vascular dysfunction in preeclampsia. Cells. 2021;**10**:11

[84] Savvidou MD, Syngelaki A, Balakitsas N, Panaiotova E, Nicolaides KH. First-trimester uterine artery Doppler examination in pregnancies complicated by gestational diabetes mellitus with or without pre-eclampsia. Ultrasound in Obstetrics & Gynecology (UOG), the official journal of the International Society of Ultrasound in Obstetrics and Gynecology. 2013;**42**(5):525-529

[85] Istrate-Ofiţeru AM, Berceanu C, Berceanu S, Busuioc CJ, Roşu GC, Diţescu D, et al. The influence of gestational diabetes mellitus (GDM) and gestational hypertension (GH) on placental morphological changes. Romanian Journal of Morphology and Embryology. 2020;**61**(2):371-384 Available from: https://pubmed.ncbi.nlm.nih.gov/33544789

[86] Downing JW, Baysinger CL, Johnson RF, Paschall RL, Shotwell MS. The effects of vasopressin and oxytocin on the fetoplacental distal stem arteriolar vascular resistance of the dual-perfused, single, isolated, human placental cotyledon. Anesthesia & Analgesia. 2016;**123**(3):698-702

[87] Stevens AD, Lumbers ER. Effects of intravenous infusions of noradrenaline into the pregnant ewe on uterine blood flow, fetal renal function, and lung liquid flow. Canadian Journal of Physiology and Pharmacology. 1995;**73**(2):202-208

[88] Christensen NJ. Plasma norepinephrine and epinephrine in untreated diabetics, during fasting and after insulin administration. Diabetes. 1974;**23**(1):1-8. DOI: 10.2337/diab.23.1.1

[89] Feng Y, Feng Q, Qu H, Song X, Hu J, Xu X, et al. Stress adaptation is associated with insulin resistance in women with gestational diabetes mellitus. Nutrition & Diabetes. 2020;**10**(1):4

[90] Levin BE. Glucose increases rat plasma norepinephrine levels by direct action on the brain. The American Journal of Physiology. 1991;**261**(6 Pt 2): R1351-R1357

[91] Walters JM, Ward GM, Barton J, Arackal R, Boston RC, Best JD, et al. The effect of norepinephrine on insulin secretion and glucose effectiveness in non-insulin-dependent diabetes. Metabolism. 1997;**46**(12):1448-1453

[92] Baron AD, Brechtel G, Johnson A, Fineberg N, Henry DP, Steinberg HO. Interactions between insulin and norepinephrine on blood pressure and insulin sensitivity. Studies in lean and obese men. Journal of Clinical Investigation. 1994;**93**(6):2453-2462. Available from: https://pubmed.ncbi.nlm.nih.gov/8200981

[93] Hiatt N, Davidson MB, Chapman LW, Sheinkopf JA. Epinephrine enhancement of potassium-stimulated immunoreactive insulin secretion. Role of beta-adrenergic receptors. Diabetes. 1978;**27**(5):550-553

[94] Yart L, Roset Bahmanyar E, Cohen M, Martinez de Tejada B. Role of the uteroplacental renin-angiotensin system in placental development and function, and its implication in the preeclampsia pathogenesis. Biomedicines. 2021;**9**(10):1332. Available from: https://pubmed.ncbi.nlm.nih.gov/34680449

[95] Kalenga MK, Thomas K, De Gasparo M, De Hertogh R. Determination of renin, angiotensin converting enzyme and angiotensin II levels in human placenta, chorion and amnion from women with pregnancy induced hypertension. Clinical Endocrinology. 1996;**44**(4):429-433. DOI: 10.1046/j.1365-2265.1996.703525.x

[96] Delforce SJ, Wang Y, Van-Aalst ME, Corbisier de Meaultsart C, Morris BJ, Broughton-Pipkin F, et al. Effect of oxygen on the expression of renin-angiotensin system components in a human trophoblast cell line. Placenta. 2016;**37**:1-6

[97] Cooper AC, Robinson G, Vinson GP, Cheung WT, Broughton PF. The localization and expression of the renin-angiotensin system in the human placenta throughout pregnancy. Placenta. 1999;**20**(5-6):467-474

[98] Kurlak LO, Mistry HD, Cindrova-Davies T, Burton GJ, Broughton PF. Human placental renin-angiotensin system in normotensive and pre-eclamptic pregnancies at high altitude and after acute hypoxia-reoxygenation insult. The Journal of Physiology. 2016;**594**(5):1327-1340

[99] Velazquez-Roman JA, Villafaña S, Lopez Sanchez P, Fernandez-Vallín E, Bobadilla Lugo RA. Effect of pregnancy and diabetes on vascular receptors for angiotensin II. Clinical and Experimental Hypertension. 2011; **33**(3):167-173

[100] Stevens AD, Lumbers ER. The effects of long-term infusions of angiotensin II into the pregnant ewe on uterine blood flow and on the fetus. Journal of Cardiovascular Pharmacology. 1999;**34**(6):824-830

[101] Samuelsson A-M, Bollano E, Mobini R, Larsson B-M, Omerovic E, Fu M, et al. Hyperinsulinemia: Effect on cardiac mass/function, angiotensin II receptor expression, and insulin signaling pathways. American Journal of Physiology—Heart and Circulatory Physiology. 2006;**291**(2):H787-H796. DOI: 10.1152/ajpheart.00974.2005

[102] Tuck ML, Bounoua F, Eslami P, Nyby MD, Eggena P, Corry DB. Insulin stimulates endogenous angiotensin II production via a mitogen-activated protein kinase pathway in vascular smooth muscle cells. Journal of Hypertension. 2004;**22**(9):1779-1785. Available from: https://journals.lww.com/jhypertension/Fulltext/2004/09000/Insulin_stimulates_endogenous_angiotensin_II.23.aspx

[103] Watanabe N, Morimoto S, Fujiwara T, Suzuki T, Taniguchi K, Mori F, et al. Prediction of gestational diabetes mellitus by soluble (pro)renin receptor during the first trimester. The Journal of Clinical Endocrinology and Metabolism. 2013;**98**(6):2528-2535

[104] Ribeiro-Oliveira A Jr, Nogueira AI, Pereira RM, Boas WWV, Dos Santos RAS, Simões e Silva AC. The renin-angiotensin system and diabetes: An update. Vascular Health and Risk Management. 2008;**4**(4):787-803. Available from: https://pubmed.ncbi.nlm.nih.gov/19065996

[105] Chu KY, Leung PS. Angiotensin II in type 2 diabetes mellitus. Current Protein & Peptide Science. 2009;**10**(1):75-84

[106] Tufiño C, Villanueva-López C, Ibarra-Barajas M, Bracho-Valdés I, Bobadilla-Lugo RA. Experimental gestational diabetes mellitus induces blunted vasoconstriction and functional changes in the rat aorta. BioMed Research International. 2014;**2014**: 329634

[107] Chen Y-P, Li J, Wang Z-N, Reichetzeder C, Xu H, Gong J, et al. Renin angiotensin aldosterone system and glycemia in pregnancy. Clinical Laboratory. 2012;**58**(5-6):527-533

[108] Chen Z-W, Tsai C-H, Pan C-T, Chou C-H, Liao C-W, Hung C-S, et al. Endothelial dysfunction in primary Aldosteronism. International Journal of Molecular Sciences. 2019;**20**(20):5214. Available from: https://pubmed.ncbi.nlm.nih.gov/31640178

[109] Zhang F, Xiao X, Liu D, Dong X, Sun J, Zhang X. Increased cord blood angiotensin II concentration is associated with decreased insulin sensitivity in the offspring of mothers with gestational diabetes mellitus. Journal of Perinatology. 2013;**33**(1):9-14. DOI: 10.1038/jp.2012.40

[110] Wei Y, Sowers JR, Nistala R, Gong H, Uptergrove GME, Clark SE, et al. Angiotensin II-induced NADPH oxidase activation impairs insulin signaling in skeletal muscle cells. Journal of Biological Chemistry. 2006;**281**(46):35137-35146. DOI: 10.1074/jbc.M601320200

[111] Olivares-Reyes JA, Arellano-Plancarte A, Castillo-Hernandez JR. Angiotensin II and the development of insulin resistance: Implications for diabetes. Molecular and Cellular Endocrinology. 2009;**302**(2):128-139

[112] Aroor AR, DeMarco VG, Jia G, Sun Z, Nistala R, Meininger GA, et al. The role of tissue renin-angiotensin-aldosterone system in the development of endothelial dysfunction and arterial stiffness. Frontiers in Endocrinology (Lausanne). 2013;**4**(October):1-7. DOI: http://journal.frontiersin.org/article/10.3389/fendo.2013.00161/abstract

[113] Hurrle S, Hsu WH. The etiology of oxidative stress in insulin resistance. Biomedical Journal. 2017;**40**(5):257-262. Available from: https://pubmed.ncbi.nlm.nih.gov/29179880

[114] Irani RA, Zhang Y, Blackwell SC, Zhou CC, Ramin SM, Kellems RE, et al. The detrimental role of angiotensin receptor agonistic autoantibodies in intrauterine growth restriction seen in preeclampsia. The Journal of Experimental Medicine. 2009; **206**(12):2809-2822

[115] Widmer RJ, Lerman A. Endothelial dysfunction and cardiovascular disease. Gobal Cardiology Science & Practice. 2014;**2014**(3):291-308. Available from: https://pubmed.ncbi.nlm.nih.gov/25780786

[116] Lerman A, Burnett JCJ. Intact and altered endothelium in regulation of vasomotion. Circulation. 1992;**86** (Suppl. 6):III12-III19

[117] Voynow JA, Kummarapurugu A. Isoprostanes and asthma. Biochimica et Biophysica Acta. 2011;**1810**(11):1091-1095

[118] Kuhn DC, Botti JJ, Cherouny PH, Demers LM. Eicosanoid production and transfer in the placenta of the diabetic pregnancy. Prostaglandins. 1990;**40**(2):205-215

[119] Wang Y, Walsh SW, Kay HH. Placental lipid peroxides and thromboxane are increased and prostacyclin is decreased in women with preeclampsia. American Journal of Obstetrics and Gynecology. 1992;**167**(4 Pt 1):946-949

[120] Ozkor MA, Quyyumi AA. Endothelium-derived hyperpolarizing factor and vascular function. Cardiology Research and Practice. 2011;**2011**:156146. Available from: https://pubmed.ncbi.nlm.nih.gov/21876822

[121] Luksha L, Luksha N, Kublickas M, Nisell H, Kublickiene K. Diverse mechanisms of endothelium-derived hyperpolarizing factor-mediated dilatation in small myometrial arteries in normal human pregnancy and preeclampsia. Biology of Reproduction. 2010;**83**(5):728-735

[122] Mokhtar SS, Vanhoutte PM, Leung SWS, Yusof MI, Wan Sulaiman WA, Mat Saad AZ, et al. Endothelium dependent hyperpolarization-type relaxation compensates for attenuated nitric oxide-mediated responses in subcutaneous arteries of diabetic patients. Nitric Oxide: Biology and Chemistry. 2016;**53**:35-44

[123] San Martín R, Sobrevia L. Gestational diabetes and the adenosine/L-arginine/nitric oxide (ALANO) pathway in human umbilical vein endothelium. Placenta. 2006;**27**(1):1-10

[124] Rafikov R, Fonseca FV, Kumar S, Pardo D, Darragh C, Elms S, et al. eNOS activation and NO function: Structural motifs responsible for the posttranslational control of endothelial nitric oxide synthase activity. The Journal of Endocrinology. 2011;**210**(3): 271-284

[125] Huang X, Liu G, Guo J, Su Z. The PI3K/AKT pathway in obesity and type 2 diabetes. International Journal of Biological Sciences. 2018;**14**(11):1483-1496. Available from: https://pubmed.ncbi.nlm.nih.gov/30263000

[126] Chae I-H, Park K-W, Kim H-S, Oh B-H. Nitric oxide-induced apoptosis is mediated by Bax/Bcl-2 gene expression, transition of cytochrome c, and activation of caspase-3 in rat vascular smooth muscle cells. Clinica Chimica Acta. 2004;**341**(1-2):83-91

[127] Tsihlis ND, Oustwani CS, Vavra AK, Jiang Q, Keefer LK, Kibbe MR. Nitric oxide inhibits vascular smooth muscle cell proliferation and neointimal hyperplasia by increasing the ubiquitination and degradation of UbcH10. Cell Biochemistry and Biophysics. 2011;**60**(1-2):89-97

[128] Yaghini FA, Song CY, Lavrentyev EN, Ghafoor HUB, Fang XR, Estes AM, et al. Angiotensin II-induced vascular smooth muscle cell migration and growth are mediated by cytochrome P450 1B1-dependent superoxide generation. Hypertens. 2010;**55**(6):1461-1467. Available from: https://pubmed.ncbi.nlm.nih.gov/20439821

[129] Tumminia A, Scalisi NM, Milluzzo A, Ettore G, Vigneri R, Sciacca L. Maternal diabetes impairs insulin and IGF-1 receptor expression and Signaling in human placenta. Frontiers in Endocrinology (Lausanne). 2021;**12**:119. Available from:. DOI: https://www.frontiersin.org/article/10.3389/fendo.2021.621680

[130] Subiabre M, Silva L, Villalobos-Labra R, Toledo F, Paublo M, López MA, et al. Maternal insulin therapy does not restore foetoplacental endothelial dysfunction in gestational diabetes mellitus. Biochimica et Biophysica Acta—Molecular Basis of Disease. 2017;**1863**(11):2987-2998

[131] Leiva A, Fuenzalida B, Barros E, Sobrevia B, Salsoso R, Sáez T, et al. Nitric oxide is a central common metabolite in vascular dysfunction associated with diseases of human pregnancy. Current Vascular Pharmacology. 2016;**14**(3):237-259

[132] Grillo MA, Lanza A, Colombatto S. Transport of amino acids through the placenta and their role. Amino Acids. 2008;**34**(4):517-523

[133] Subiabre M, Villalobos-Labra R, Silva L, Fuentes G, Toledo F, Sobrevia L. Role of insulin, adenosine, and adipokine receptors in the foetoplacental vascular dysfunction in gestational diabetes mellitus. Biochim Biophys Acta—Molecular Basis of Disease. 2020;**1866**(2):165370. DOI: 10.1016/j.bbadis.2018.12.021

[134] Ballard-Croft C, Locklar AC, Keith BJ, Mentzer RMJ, Lasley RD. Oxidative stress and adenosine A1 receptor activation differentially modulate subcellular cardiomyocyte MAPKs. American Journal of Physiology. Heart and Circulatory Physiology. 2008;**294**(1):H263-H271

[135] Guzmán-Gutiérrez E, Westermeier F, Salomón C, González M, Pardo F, Leiva A, et al. Insulin-increased L-arginine transport requires A(2A) adenosine receptors activation in human umbilical vein endothelium. PLoS One. 2012;**7**(7):e41705

[136] Farías M, Puebla C, Westermeier F, Jo MJ, Pastor-Anglada M, Casanello P, et al. Nitric oxide reduces SLC29A1 promoter activity and adenosine transport involving transcription factor complex hCHOP-C/EBPalpha in human umbilical vein endothelial cells from gestational diabetes. Cardiovascular Research. 2010;**86**(1):45-54

[137] Westermeier F, Salomón C, González M, Puebla C, Guzmán-Gutiérrez E, Cifuentes F, et al. Insulin

restores gestational diabetes mellitus-reduced adenosine transport involving differential expression of insulin receptor isoforms in human umbilical vein endothelium. Diabetes. 2011;**60**(6): 1677-1687

[138] Feoktistov I, Goldstein AE, Ryzhov S, Zeng D, Belardinelli L, Voyno-Yasenetskaya T, et al. Differential expression of adenosine receptors in human endothelial cells. Circulation Research. 2002;**90**(5):531-538. DOI: 10.1161/01.RES.0000012203.21416.14

[139] Razak AA, Leach L, Ralevic V. Impaired vasocontractile responses to adenosine in chorionic vessels of human term placenta from pregnant women with pre-existing and gestational diabetes. Diabetes & Vascular Disease Research. 2018;**15**(6):528-540

[140] Baldea I, Teacoe I, Olteanu DE, Vaida-Voievod C, Clichici A, Sirbu A, et al. Effects of different hypoxia degrees on endothelial cell cultures-time course study. Mechanisms of Ageing and Development. 2018;**172**:45-50

[141] Volpe CMO, Villar-Delfino PH, dos Anjos PMF, Nogueira-Machado JA. Cellular death, reactive oxygen species (ROS) and diabetic complications. Cell Death and Disease. 2018;**9**(2):119. DOI: 10.1038/s41419-017-0135-z

[142] Sada K, Nishikawa T, Kukidome D, Yoshinaga T, Kajihara N, Sonoda K, et al. Hyperglycemia induces cellular hypoxia through production of mitochondrial ROS followed by suppression of aquaporin-1. PLoS One. 2016;**11**(7):e0158619. Available from: DOI: 10.1371/journal.pone.0158619

[143] Sobrevia L, Valero P, Grismaldo A, Villalobos-Labra R, Pardo F, Subiabre M, et al. Mitochondrial dysfunction in the fetoplacental unit in gestational diabetes mellitus. Biochimica et Biophysica Acta: Molecular Basis of Disease. 2020;**1866**(12):165948. DOI: 10.1016/j.bbadis.2020.165948

[144] Fisher JJ, Vanderpeet CL, Bartho LA, McKeating DR, Cuffe JSM, Holland OJ, et al. Mitochondrial dysfunction in placental trophoblast cells experiencing gestational diabetes mellitus. The Journal of Physiology. 2021;**599**(4):1291-1305

[145] Lappas M, Mitton A, Permezel M. In response to oxidative stress, the expression of inflammatory cytokines and antioxidant enzymes are impaired in placenta, but not adipose tissue, of women with gestational diabetes. The Journal of Endocrinology. 2010;**204**(1): 75-84

[146] Brown GC. Nitric oxide and mitochondrial respiration. Biochimica et Biophysica Acta. 1999;**1411**(2-3): 351-369

[147] Eppel D, Feichtinger M, Lindner T, Kotzaeridi G, Rosicky I, Yerlikaya-Schatten G, et al. Association between maternal triglycerides and disturbed glucose metabolism in pregnancy. Acta Diabetologica. 2021;**58**(4):459-465

[148] Dubé M-C, Morrisset A-S, Tchernof A, Weisnagel SJ. Cord blood C-peptide levels relate to the metabolic profile of women with and without gestational diabetes. Acta Obstetricia et Gynecologica Scandinavica. 2012;**91**(12):1469-1473. DOI: 10.1111/aogs.12005

[149] Eslamian L, Akbari S, Marsoosi V, Jamal A. Association between fetal overgrowth and metabolic parameters in cord blood of newborns of women with GDM. Minerva Medica. 2013;**104**(3):317-324

[150] Son GH, Kwon JY, Kim YH, Park YW. Maternal serum triglycerides as predictive factors for large-for-gestational age newborns in women

with gestational diabetes mellitus. Acta Obstetricia et Gynecologica Scandinavica. 2010;**89**(5):700-704

[151] Herrera E, Ortega-Senovilla H. Disturbances in lipid metabolism in diabetic pregnancy—Are these the cause of the problem? Best Practice & Research Clinical Endocrinology & Metabolism. 2010;**24**(4):515-525. DOI: 10.1016/j.beem.2010.05.006

[152] Abbassi-Ghanavati M, Greer LG, Cunningham FG. Pregnancy and laboratory studies: A reference table for clinicians. Obstetrics and Gynecology. 2009;**114**(6):1326-1331

[153] Villafan-Bernal JR, Acevedo-Alba M, Reyes-Pavon R, Diaz-Parra GA, Lip-Sosa DL, Vazquez-Delfin HI, et al. Plasma levels of free fatty acids in women with gestational diabetes and its intrinsic and extrinsic determinants: Systematic review and meta-analysis. Journal of Diabetes Research. 2019;**2019**:7098470. Available from: https://pubmed.ncbi.nlm.nih.gov/31531374

[154] Bomba-Opon D, Wielgos M, Szymanska M, Bablok L. Effects of free fatty acids on the course of gestational diabetes mellitus. Neuro Endocrinology Letters. 2006;**27**(1-2):277-280

[155] Kajikawa M, Higashi Y. Triglycerides and endothelial function: Molecular biology to clinical perspective. Current Opinion in Lipidology. 2019;**30**(5):364-369. Available from: https://journals.lww.com/co-lipidology/Fulltext/2019/10000/Triglycerides_and_endothelial_function__molecular.3.aspx

[156] Milosavljevic D, Kontush A, Griglio S, Le Naour G, Thillet J, Chapman MJ. VLDL-induced triglyceride accumulation in human macrophages is mediated by modulation of LPL lipolytic activity in the absence of change in LPL mass. Biochimica et Biophysica Acta. 2003;**1631**(1):51-60

[157] Wang L, Gill R, Pedersen TL, Higgins LJ, Newman JW, Rutledge JC. Triglyceride-rich lipoprotein lipolysis releases neutral and oxidized FFAs that induce endothelial cell inflammation. Journal of Lipid Research. 2009;**50**(2):204-213

[158] Castillo-Castrejon M, Powell TL. Placental nutrient transport in gestational diabetic pregnancies. Frontiers in Endocrinology (Lausanne). 2017;**8**:306. Available from:. DOI: https://www.frontiersin.org/article/10.3389/fendo.2017.00306

[159] Ericsson A, Hamark B, Powell TL, Jansson T. Glucose transporter isoform 4 is expressed in the syncytiotrophoblast of first trimester human placenta. Human Reproduction. 2005;**20**(2):521-530

[160] Illsley NP. Glucose transporters in the human placenta. Placenta. 2000;**21**(1):14-22

[161] Borges MH, Pullockaran J, Catalano P, Baumann MU, Illsley NP. Human placental GLUT1 glucose transporter expression and the fetal insulin-like growth factor axis in pregnancies complicated by diabetes. Biochimica et Biophysica Acta. Molecular Basis of Disease. 2019;**1865**(9):2411-2419

[162] James-Allan LB, Arbet J, Teal SB, Powell TL, Jansson T. Insulin stimulates GLUT4 trafficking to the Syncytiotrophoblast basal plasma membrane in the human placenta. The Journal of Clinical Endocrinology and Metabolism. 2019;**104**(9):4225-4238

[163] Díaz P, Dimasuay KG, Koele-Schmidt L, Jang B, Barbour LA, Jansson T, et al. Glyburide treatment in gestational diabetes is associated with increased placental glucose transporter

1 expression and higher birth weight. Placenta. 2017;**57**:52-59

[164] Stanirowski PJ, Szukiewicz D, Pyzlak M, Abdalla N, Sawicki W, Cendrowski K. Impact of pre-gestational and gestational diabetes mellitus on the expression of glucose transporters GLUT-1, GLUT-4 and GLUT-9 in human term placenta. Endocrine [Internet]. 2017;**55**(3):799-808. Available from: https://pubmed.ncbi.nlm.nih.gov/27981520

[165] Gaither K, Quraishi AN, Illsley NP. Diabetes alters the expression and activity of the human placental GLUT1 glucose transporter. The Journal of Clinical Endocrinology and Metabolism. 1999;**84**(2):695-701

[166] Illsley NP, Sellers MC, Wright RL. Glycaemic regulation of glucose transporter expression and activity in the human placenta. Placenta. 1998;**19**(7):517-524

[167] Hahn T, Barth S, Graf R, Engelmann M, Beslagic D, Reul JM, et al. Placental glucose transporter expression is regulated by glucocorticoids. The Journal of Clinical Endocrinology and Metabolism. 1999;**84**(4):1445-1452

[168] Challier JC, Hauguel S, Desmaizieres V. Effect of insulin on glucose uptake and metabolism in the human placenta. The Journal of Clinical Endocrinology and Metabolism. 1986;**62**(5):803-807

[169] Kamana KCS, Shakya ZH. Gestational diabetes mellitus and macrosomia: A literature review. Annals of Nutrition & Metabolism. 2015;**66**:14-20

Chapter 8

Gestational Diabetes Mellitus and Maternal Microbiome Alterations

Dalia Rafat

Abstract

The maternal microbiome has been identified as a critical driver for a variety of important mother and child health outcomes. Studies have demonstrated changes in maternal microbiome during pregnancy. These changes may have an impact on the maternal metabolic profile, play a role in pregnancy problems, and contribute to the metabolic and immunological health of the offspring. Gestational diabetes mellitus is a major challenge for prenatal healthcare providers, not only because of the negative short and long-term effects on the mother's and baby's health, but also because its aetiology has been poorly understood till now. The developing link between maternal microbiome and metabolic disorders in pregnancy can be offered as a new target in their prevention and treatment, as well as in reducing their negative health outcomes; however, there has been very little research done on this. Diabetes' impact on site-specific maternal microbiome alterations during pregnancy is similarly poorly understood. Given the rising prevalence of diabetes in pregnancy and the potential importance of the maternal microbiome, more research is needed to understand and rigorously examine how metabolic disorders in pregnancy affect the pregnancy-associated microbiome, as well as whether these microbial alterations affect the health of the mother and her offspring.

Keywords: pregnancy, gut microbiota, vaginal microbiota, oral microbiota, gestational diabetes mellitus

1. Introduction

The human body harbors complex community of microorganisms over different sites in the body [1]. Numerous microorganisms live in the human body and maintain a stable symbiotic relationship with the host, which is essential for human health. These unique microbial communities residing on and in the human body comprise "Human microbiome". The Human Microbiome Project [1], launched to demonstrate the human microbial flora and its association with human health, characterized the microbial communities residing over five areas in the body: oral cavity, nasal cavity, skin, gastrointestinal tract and genitourinary system. They found that more than 10,000 microbial species harbor the human body and successfully identified around 81–99% of genera constituting the human ecosystem [1].

The significance of the human microbiome in preserving health is becoming increasingly evident, and it may potentially guard against unfavorable health outcomes by stimulating or suppressing both genetic and environmental risk factors. The gut microbiome, for example, has been linked to the body's immune system, since it protects against various invading bacteria [2]. Likewise, the healthy vaginal microbiome has an important role in the prevention of various cervicovaginal infections [3]. Besides a variety of diseases have been linked to an imbalance in the human microbiota. The use of human microbiome as disease biomarkers has become a promising strategy [4, 5]. Studies have discovered that using microbiome composition and alterations to diagnose diseases has a lot of promise [6].

2. Pregnancy and human microbiome

Women underwent a variety of physiological changes throughout pregnancy. During pregnancy, the maternal body habitat microbiome composition changes as well [7, 8]. The maternal microbiome has been recognized as a key determinant of a range of important maternal and child health outcomes, and together with perinatal factors influences the infant microbiome [9].

The microbiome alterations and disturbances during pregnancy and neonatal life has received great interest in recent years owing to the crucial role it plays in reproductive health. These changes may have an impact on the maternal metabolic profile, play a role in pregnancy complications, and contribute to the metabolic and immunological health of the offspring [9], implying that microbial communities' interactions with pregnant women are crucial.

3. Gestational diabetes mellitus and human microbiome

Diabetes and related metabolic disorders are rapidly increasing among pregnant women throughout the world [10, 11]. Gestational Diabetes Mellitus (GDM) is a major challenge for obstetric practice not only because of the adverse short and long term fetomaternal health consequences but also because of its improperly understood etiology till now. Current prevention strategies focusing on changes to diet and physical activity have resulted in limited success leading to an urgent need for alternative strategies.

The significance of the microbiome in many physiological processes involved in health and the development of various diseases is still unknown. Due to increased inflammation, insulin resistance, and weight gain in women with GDM, it has been postulated that the physiological adaptation of the microbial pattern seen in pregnancy is disrupted in women with metabolic illnesses, such as GDM [8, 12].

Microbiome and its alterations at various body sites has been demonstrated to influence metabolic disorders by a number of researchers. As only few scant studies are done on microbiome's complexity of different body compartments in GDM [5, 13], their interactions and exact role in the pathogenesis of GDM is still not clear. Some researchers have indicated that GDM has no clear effect on the microbial composition [14] while others have found that the microbiota of GDM patients and normal pregnant women differs significantly [5, 13, 15].

Studies have demonstrated that microbiome of different body compartments like gut/oral/vaginal microbiome influences gestational development and metabolic disorders. It however is still not clear whether there is an interaction between the microbiome of the different compartments and their role in GDM pathogenesis.

3.1 GDM and gut microbiome

Human gut microbiome is becoming more well acknowledged as key contributor to host metabolism and health [16]. The maternal gut microbiota changes dramatically during pregnancy [8] and has been linked to a variety of adverse pregnancy outcomes, including obesity, gestational hypertension and GDM [17]. Researchers are exploring the gut immune system as a new therapeutic target for systemic inflammation in insulin resistance. As a result, the gut microbiota has been the focus of several investigations on GDM and several recent investigations have found specific changes in gut microbiome between pregnant women with and without GDM [5, 18–22]. According to current theories, the proposed pathogenesis of insulin resistance due to dysbiosis of intestinal microbiota; include influencing inflammatory responses [23], boosting fat accumulation [24], controlling bile acid metabolism [25], and regulating amino acid metabolism [26].

Understanding the gut microbiota's alterations will not only help us better understand GDM pathogenesis but will also promote prospective preventive approaches for GDM based on gut microbiota modification. Although various studies have linked maternal gut microbiota dysbiosis to GDM, the exact potential role of gut microbiota in the etiology of GDM is still unclear. Future large-sampled well-designed studies are required to elucidate the role of gut bacterial dysbiosis in the pathogenesis of GDM, and in exploring gut microbiota-targeted biomarkers as potential predictors of GDM.

3.2 GDM and vaginal microbiome

The healthy vaginal microbiome has an important role in the prevention of bacterial vaginosis, vaginal candidiasis, and other cervicovaginal infections [3]. During pregnancy, there is a change in the structure of the vaginal microbiome [7, 27], which contributes in increasing the presence and stabilization of Lactobacillus in the vaginal microbiome [27, 28]. Besides preventing bacterial invasion, the vaginal microbiome has been postulated to play vital role in timing parturition, hormone secretion and, importantly, seedling of infant microbiome during birth.

Emerging studies have reported link between the vaginal microbiome and metabolic illnesses such GDM [20, 29]. Studies have demonstrated increased inflammatory cytokine expression in GDM, together with the presence of potentially pathogenic bacteria, indicating a dysbiotic profile of the vaginal microbiome [20].

Researchers have speculated on the role of the vaginal microbiota in pregnancy outcomes, which have been shown to have a negative impact on neonatal and infant health, as well as the association of the vaginal microbiome with both health and disease states, but there are few studies to validate these speculations. According to the limited scarce studies on this subject, pregnant women with hyperglycemia have a greater prevalence of vaginal infections, and both hyperglycemia and an aberrant vaginal dysbiosis are linked to poor fetomaternal outcomes [12, 20, 29]. Exploring the vaginal microbiome alterations of women with GDM and its relationship to adverse pregnancy outcomes could help in the early detection and treatment of dysbiotic alterations that could lead to poor maternal and neonatal outcomes.

3.3 GDM and oral microbiome

The oral microbiome has been proposed in the development of a variety of diseases, but its link to GDM is still a mystery. Recent studies have shown substantial changes in the oral microbiota between GDM and non GDM patients in pregnancy and puerperium [30] indicating potential role of the oral microbiome as noninvasive GDM biomarkers.

Numerous studies have demonstrated a link between GDM and periodontitis [31, 32]. The incidence of GDM has been reported to be higher in people with periodontitis. Periodontal infection has been linked to an increased risk of GDM via disrupting endocrine metabolism and blood glucose regulation [33], although it is unclear whether the relationships between these two diseases are caused by microbiome alterations.

Future large scale studies are required to analyze the oral microbiome of GDM patients and healthy pregnant women to see whether there are any links between GDM and two main oral diseases: dental caries and chronic periodontitis. Also studies are required to find appropriate oral microbial markers for constructing GDM classification models and establish simple and noninvasive techniques for supplementary diagnosis and daily GDM follow-up.

4. Conclusion

There is potential importance of the maternal microbiome for maternal and infant health. Pregnancy-related changes to the maternal microbiota are evolutionarily adaptive to promote the nutrition and development of the mother and fetus during pregnancy, and the child after birth. The developing link between maternal microbiota and metabolic disorders in pregnancy can be offered as a new target in their prevention and treatment, as well as in reducing their negative maternal and neonatal outcomes, however there has been very little research done on this. Lack of robust research on the impact of diabetes on the maternal microbiota during pregnancy is also a problem. Large longitudinal cohort studies of racially and ethnically diverse mother-child dyads are required to rigorously examine how hyperglycemia in pregnancy modifies the pregnancy-associated microbiota and the mother-to-newborn vertical transfer of microbiota, and to consider whether these microbial alterations affect the health of the mother and her offspring, and if these microbial alterations can ultimately be targeted for interventions that improve public health.

Author details

Dalia Rafat
Department of Obstetrics and Gynaecology, Jawaharlal Nehru Medical College, AMU, Aligarh, UP, India

*Address all correspondence to: drdaliarafat.16@gmail.com

References

[1] The Human Microbiome Project Consortium. Structure, function and diversity of the healthy human microbiome. Nature. 2012;**486**:207-214

[2] Wardwell LH, Huttenhower C, Garrett WS. Current concepts of the intestinal microbiota and pathogenesis of infection. Current Infectious Disease Reports. 2011;**13**:28-34

[3] Donders GG, Dekeersmaeker A, Vereecken A, Van Bulck B, Spitz B. Pathogenesis of abnormal vaginal bacterial flora. American Journal of Obstetrics and Gynecology. 2000;**182**:872-878

[4] Wang J, Jia Z, Zhang B, Peng L, Zhao F. Tracing the accumulation of *in vivo* human oral microbiota elucidates microbial community dynamics at the gateway to the GI tract. Gut. 2019;**69**: 1355-1356

[5] Wang J, Zheng J, Shi W, Du N, Xu X, Zhang Y, et al. Dysbiosis of maternal and neonatal microbiota associated with gestational diabetes mellitus. Gut. 2018;**67**:1614-1625

[6] Martinez KB, Leone V, Chang EB. Microbial metabolites in health and disease: Navigating the unknown in search of function. The Journal of Biological Chemistry. 2017;**292**: 8553-8559

[7] Aagaard K, Riehle K, Ma J, Segata N, Mistretta T-A, Coarfa C, et al. A metagenomic approach to characterization of the vaginal microbiome signature in pregnancy. PLoS One. 2012;**7**(6):e36466

[8] Koren O, Goodrich Julia K, Cullender Tyler C, Spor A, Laitinen K, Kling Bäckhed H, et al. Host remodeling of the gut microbiome and metabolic changes during pregnancy. Cell. 2012;**150**(3):470-480

[9] Laker RC, Wlodek ME, Connelly JJ, Yan Z. Epigenetic origins of metabolic disease: The impact of the maternal condition to the offspring epigenome and later health consequences. Food Science and Human Wellness. 2013;**2**(1):1-11

[10] Anna V, van der Ploeg HP, Cheung NW, Huxley RR, Bauman AE. Sociodemographic correlates of the increasing trend in prevalence of gestational diabetes mellitus in a large population of women between 1995 and 2005. Diabetes Care. 2008;**31**(12): 2288-2293

[11] Zhu Y, Zhang C. Prevalence of gestational diabetes and risk of progression to type 2 diabetes: A global perspective. Current Diabetes Reports. 2016;**16**(1):7

[12] Taddei CR, Cortez RV, Mattar R, Torloni MR, Daher S. Microbiome in normal and pathological pregnancies: A literature overview. American Journal of Reproductive Immunology. 2018;**80**:e12993

[13] Acuna J, Cohavy O, Solt I, Reeder J, Kim M, Lebovics I, et al. Preliminary observations on the microbial phylogeny of the oral, vaginal, and rectal microbiome in gestational diabetes and healthy pregnancies Am. J. Obstetrics and Gynecology. 2011;**204**:S109-S110

[14] Hasan S, Aho V, Pereira P, Paulin L, Koivusalo SB, Auvinen P, et al. Gut microbiome in gestational diabetes: A cross-sectional study of mothers and offspring 5 years postpartum. Acta Obstetricia et Gynecologica Scandinavica. 2018;**97**:38-46

[15] Crusell MKW, Brink LR, Nielsen T, Allin KH, Hansen T, Damm P, et al. Gestational diabetes and the human salivary microbiota: A longitudinal

study during pregnancy and postpartum. BMC Pregnancy and Childbirth. 2020;**20**:69

[16] Le Chatelier E, Nielsen T, Qin J, Prifti E, Hildebrand F, Falony G, et al. Richness of human gut microbiome correlates with metabolic markers. Nature. 2013;**500**:541-546

[17] Winer DA, Luck H, Tsai S, Winer S. The intestinal immune system in obesity and insulin resistance. Cell Metabolism. 2016;**23**:413-426

[18] Kuang Y-S, Lu J-H, Li S-H, Li J-H, Yuan M-Y, He J-R, et al. Connections between the human gut microbiome and gestational diabetes mellitus. Gigascience. 2017;**6**:1-12

[19] Mokkala K, Houttu N, Vahlberg T, Munukka E, Rönnemaa T, Laitinen K. Gut microbiota aberrations precede diagnosis of gestational diabetes mellitus. Acta Diabetologica. 2017a;**54**:1147-1149

[20] Cortez RV, Taddei CR, Sparvoli LG, Ângelo AGS, Padilha M, Mattar R, et al. Microbiome and its relation to gestational diabetes. Endocrine. 2018;**64**:254-264

[21] Crusell MKW, Hansen TH, Nielsen T, Allin KH, Rühlemann MC, Damm P, et al. Gestational diabetes is associated with change in the gut microbiota composition in third trimester of pregnancy and postpartum. Microbiome. 2018;**6**:89

[22] Ye G, Zhang L, Wang M, Chen Y, Gu S, Wang K, et al. The gut microbiota in women suffering from gestational diabetes mellitus with the failure of glycemic control by lifestyle modification. Journal Diabetes Research. 2019;**2019**:1-12

[23] Cani PD, Delzenne NM. The role of the gut microbiota in energy metabolism and metabolic disease. Current Pharmaceutical Design. 2009;**15**: 1546-1558

[24] Bäckhed F, Ding H, Wang T, Hooper LV, Koh GY, Nagy A, et al. The gut microbiota as an environmental factor that regulates fat storage. Proceeding of the National Acadamy of Sciences USA. 2004;**101**:15718-15723

[25] Gu Y, Wang X, Li J, Zhang Y, Zhong H, Liu R, et al. Analyses of gut microbiota and plasma bile acids enable stratification of patients for antidiabetic treatment. Nature Communications. 2017;**8**:1785

[26] Koh A, Molinaro A, Ståhlman M, Khan MT, Schmidt C, Mannerås-Holm L, et al. Microbially produced imidazole propionate impairs insulin signaling through mTORC1. Cell. 2018;**175**: 947-961.e17

[27] Romero R, Hassan SS, Gajer P, Tarca AL, Fadrosh DW, Nikita L, et al. The composition and stability of the vaginal microbiota of normal pregnant women is different from that of non-pregnant women. Microbiome. 2014;**2**:4

[28] Nasioudis D, Forney LJ, Schneider GM, Gliniewicz K, France M, Boester A, et al. Influence of pregnancy history on the vaginal microbiome of pregnant women in their first trimester. Scientific Reports. 2017;**7**:10201

[29] Rafat D, Singh S, Nawab T, Khan F, Khan AU, Khalid S. Association of vaginal dysbiosis and gestational diabetes mellitus with adverse perinatal outcomes. International Journal of Gynecology & Obstetrics. 2021;**00**:1-9. DOI: 10.1002/ijgo.13945

[30] Crusell MKW, Brink LR, Nielsen T, Allin KH, Hansen T, Damm P, et al. Gestational diabetes and the human salivary microbiota: A longitudinal study during pregnancy and post-partum. BMC Pregnancy and Childbirth. 2020;**20**:69

[31] Belstrom D, Paster BJ, Fiehn NE, Bardow A, Holmstrup P. Salivary bacterial fingerprints of established oral disease revealed by the Human Oral Microbe Identification using Next Generation Sequencing technique. Journal of Oral Microbiology. 2016;**8**:30170

[32] Graziani F, Gennai S, Solini A, Petrini M. A systematic review and meta- analysis of epidemiologic observational evidence on the effect of periodontitis on diabetes an update of the EFP-AAP review. Journal of Clinical Periodontology. 2018;**45**:167-e187

[33] Gumus P, Ozcaka O, Ceyhan-Ozturk B, Akcali A, Lappin DF, Buduneli N. Evaluation of biochemical parameters and local and systemic levels of osteoactive and B-cell stimulatory factors in gestational diabetes in the presence or absence of gingivitis. Journal of Periodontology. 2015;**86**:387-e397

Chapter 9

Future Risks for Children Born to Mothers with Gestational Diabetes: Elucidation Using the Cell Model Approach

Ritsuko Kawaharada and Akio Nakamura

Abstract

A number of studies have shown that foetal nutritional status significantly impacts an unborn child's long-term health. The developmental origins of health and disease (DOHaD) hypothesis proposes that if a child is undernourished in the foetal period, the child will develop diabetes and hypertension in the future if adequate nutrition is given after birth. Moreover, hyperglycaemia (e.g. gestational diabetes mellitus [GDM]) experienced during foetal life can reportedly cause various complications in children. As diabetes is increasing worldwide, so is GDM, and many studies have been conducted using GDM animal models and GDM cell lines. We examined the effects of streptozotocin-induced diabetes, particularly on the heart of offspring, in rat GDM animal models. We also analysed primary cardiomyocyte cultures isolated from these GDM rats and found that insulin signalling was inhibited in GDM cells, as in the GDM animal models, by increased advanced glycation end products. Furthermore, the effect of eicosapentaenoic acid during pregnancy has been reported in GDM animal models and cells, and the findings indicated the importance of nutritional management for GDM during pregnancy.

Keywords: developmental origins of health and disease, fetus, high glucose, hyperglycaemia, advanced glycation end products, eicosapentaenoic acid

1. Introduction

Several studies have shown that foetal nutritional status has a significant impact on an unborn child's long-term health. Barker et al. found that areas with high neonatal mortality between 1921 and 1925 had higher cardiovascular mortality between 1969 and 1978 [1]. Barker et al. later reported that low birth weight correlated with glucose intolerance and cardiovascular disorders [2, 3]. Furthermore, they also proposed the Barker theory that "prenatal undernutrition increases the risk of lifestyle-related diseases in adulthood" [4]. Later, Gluckman and Hanson proposed the developmental origins of health and disease (DOHaD) hypothesis, which states that predisposition to lifestyle-related diseases is shaped by gene–environment interactions during fertilisation, embryonic development, foetal life, and infancy and that excessive nutrition after birth leads to the development of diabetes and hypertension (**Figures 1** and **2**) [5, 6].

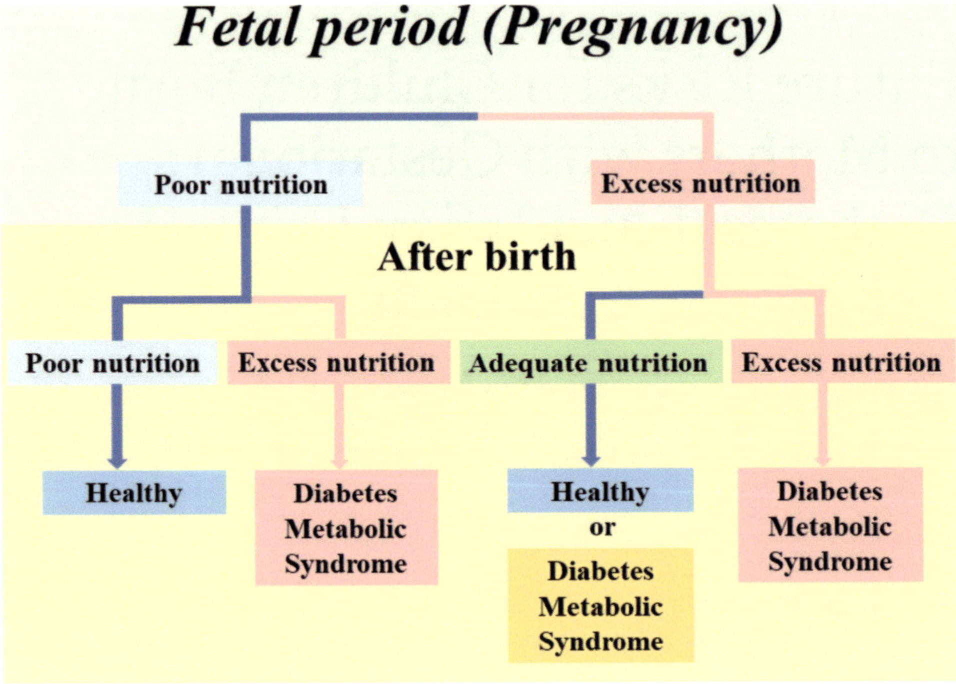

Figure 1.
Foetal nutritional status has a major impact on postnatal health. It has been shown that even if the mother is undernourished during pregnancy, if the child is well nourished after birth, the child will develop diabetes and metabolic syndrome in the future. This has been defined as the developmental origin of health and disease (DOHaD) hypothesis. By contrast, GDM, an excessive nutrition (high glucose) environment during pregnancy, similarly increases the child's risk of developing diabetes and metabolic syndrome in the future. Many studies have reported that nutritional status during pregnancy has a significant impact on the health of the child.

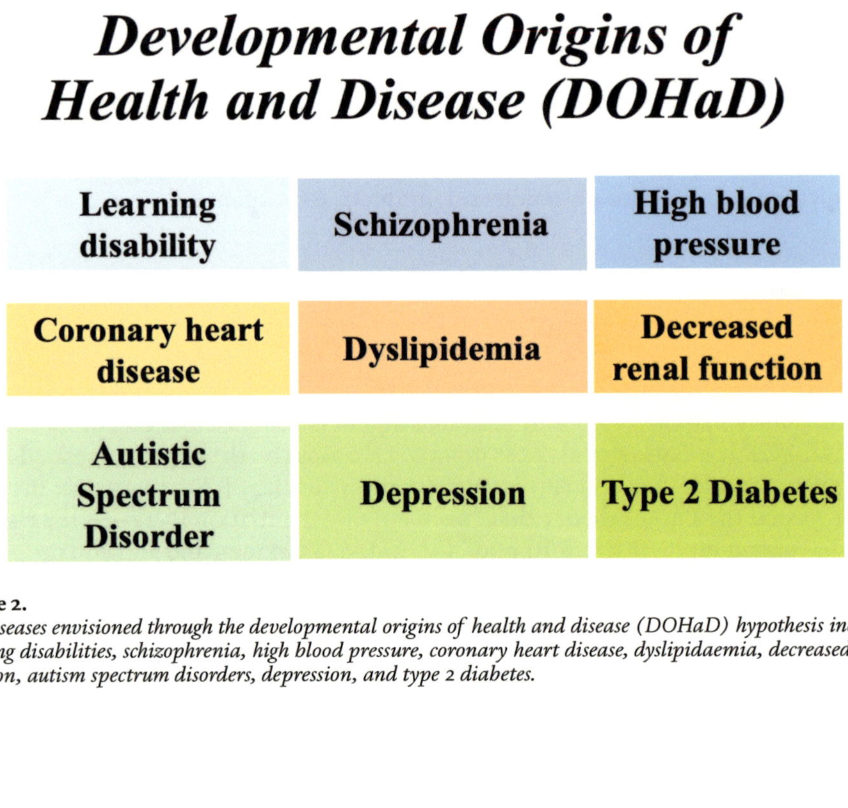

Figure 2.
The diseases envisioned through the developmental origins of health and disease (DOHaD) hypothesis include learning disabilities, schizophrenia, high blood pressure, coronary heart disease, dyslipidaemia, decreased renal function, autism spectrum disorders, depression, and type 2 diabetes.

DOI: http://dx.doi.org/10.5772/intechopen.100117

This hypothesis is also supported by many epidemiological studies, which now clearly show that low birth weight increases the risk of developing a diverse array of diseases, such as coronary artery disease, hypertension, stroke, diabetes, obesity, and metabolic syndrome. One example is the findings during the Dutch winter famine, wherein calorie intake had been temporarily lowered to 700 kcal/day for six months in 1944 due to the food embargo in the Netherlands during World War II. Children born during this period exhibited an increased risk of developing various diseases in adulthood, including glucose intolerance, lipid disorders, and ischemic heart disease. Moreover, during the starvation caused by China's Great Leap Forward policy, those born during this period reportedly had an increased risk of type 2 diabetes and hypertension [7, 8]. Highly accurate and detailed birth record data such as birth weight, postnatal weight, and placental size were recorded at the University of Helsinki Hospital from 1934 to 1944. Barker and his colleagues analysed the records and found that children with low birth weight were more likely to develop myocardial infarction, diabetes, and hypertension, as well as cognitive decline and depression in the future [9–12].

It is very difficult to prove a causal relationship between these foetal intrauterine environmental factors and their effects on the development of postnatal health and illness. However, in recent years, basic research using pregnant animal models as well as cell models are gradually clarifying the underlying molecular mechanism. In this chapter, we will introduce the findings on the effects of overnutrition, as represented by gestational diabetes mellitus (GDM), on animal offspring, rather than discuss findings from the perspective of undernutrition during the foetal period, which has already been extensively studied.

The structure of this paper is as follows: the introduction section describes the DOHaD theory and provides a description on the increasing number of diabetic patients worldwide; Section 2 provides an overview of gestational diabetes; Section 3 describes the use of GDM animal models; Section 4 describes studies using hyperglycaemia cell models; and Section 5 describes the latest research on drug and diet therapy for GDM.

2. Gestational diabetes mellitus

The International Diabetes Federation (IDF) estimates that the global diabetes population continues to increase with 463 million people being pre-diabetic in 2019 with a projected increase of up to 578 million by 2030. In addition, one in six women will develop abnormal glucose metabolism during pregnancy. The IDF has identified women with diabetes as a key challenge, with measures to improve the control of all types of diabetes being needed [13]. The prevalence of type 1 and type 2 diabetes in women of childbearing age is increasing, affecting about 1% of all pregnancies. Prevention is also important because of the increasing costs of diabetes care. Babies with extremely low or high birth weight are at high risk of diabetes [10]; therefore, nutritional management during pregnancy is important. Furthermore, inadequate glycaemic control in early pregnancy is associated with increased rates of congenital malformations, spontaneous abortions, stillbirths, and perinatal mortality [14–18]. It may also be associated with various pregnancy complications as well as neurodevelopmental disorders in the offspring. Similarly, long-term problems in the offspring due to insulin resistance may increase the risk of cardiovascular disease, hypertension, and diabetes mellitus (metabolic syndrome).

GDM is one of the most frequent complications of pregnancy, with an increasing rate [19, 20]. The prevalence of GDM varies in direct proportion to the prevalence of type 2 diabetes and is higher among Hispanic, African American, Native American, Asian or Pacific Islander, and South Mediterranean women [21, 22]. It also varies by maternal age and diagnostic criteria [23, 24]. Since 2010, the international Association for the Study of Diabetes and Pregnancy (IADPSG) has tightened the criteria for the diagnosis of GDM, based on the 2008 Hyperglycemia and Adverse Pregnancy Outcomes (HAPO) study [25]. The reason for this was that the HAPO study reported a higher risk of macrosomia in newborn born to mothers with high blood glucose levels, even though GDM was not diagnosed using the previous criteria [26]. As a result, many GDM patients have been identified. The HAPO study was a large observational study of approximately 25,000 pregnant women with impaired glucose tolerance conducted in 15 centres across 9 countries; the correlation between blood glucose levels was examined at 24–32 weeks' gestation with various pregnancy complications [27]. The endpoints of the diagnostic criteria for GDM were perinatal factors (heavy-for-dates infants, first caesarean section, neonatal hypoglycaemia, and hyperinsulinemia in the infant). The results showed that these perinatal complications were significantly associated with maternal blood glucose levels, even after adjusting for confounding factors such as maternal obesity. Furthermore, many epidemiological studies have shown that children born with GDM are associated with future development of noncommunicable diseases (NCDs) such as obesity and diabetes. Clausen et al. reported that the hyperglycaemic environment in utero and genetic background are associated with the future development of diabetes in children [28]. Sugihara et al. reported that infants born with macrosomia were also associated with childhood diabetes compared with low and normal birth weight [29].

Maternal undernutrition as well as GDM in an overnutrition environment are associated with the development of NCDs in future infants, indicating the importance of nutritional management during pregnancy (**Figures 3** and **4**) [29].

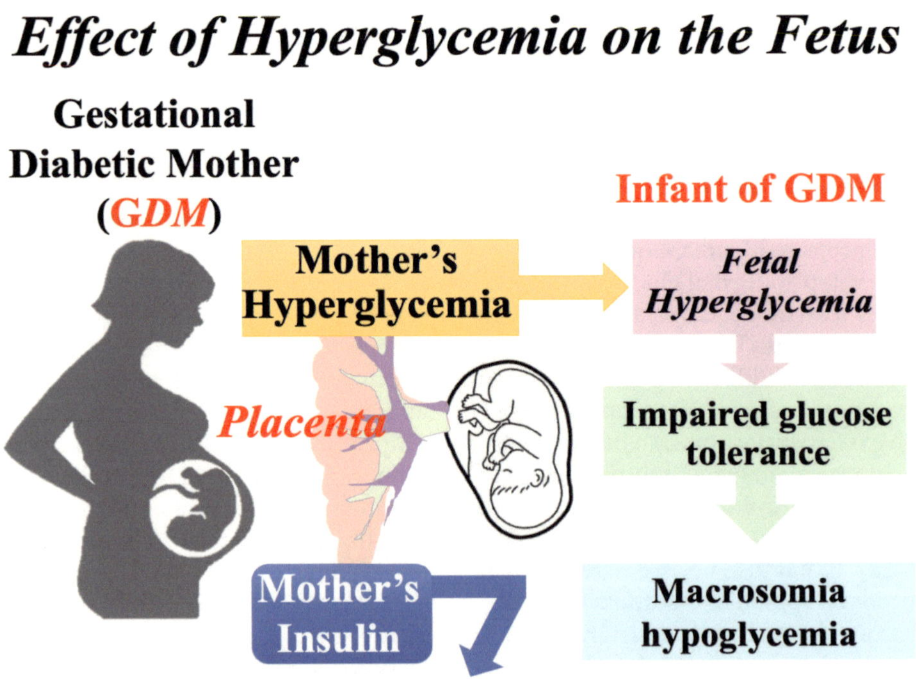

Figure 3.
Similar to GDM, if the mother is hyperglycaemic, the foetus becomes exposed to hyperglycaemia. If hyperglycaemia persists, the foetus will develop insulin resistance and complications such as macrosomia and hypoglycaemia.

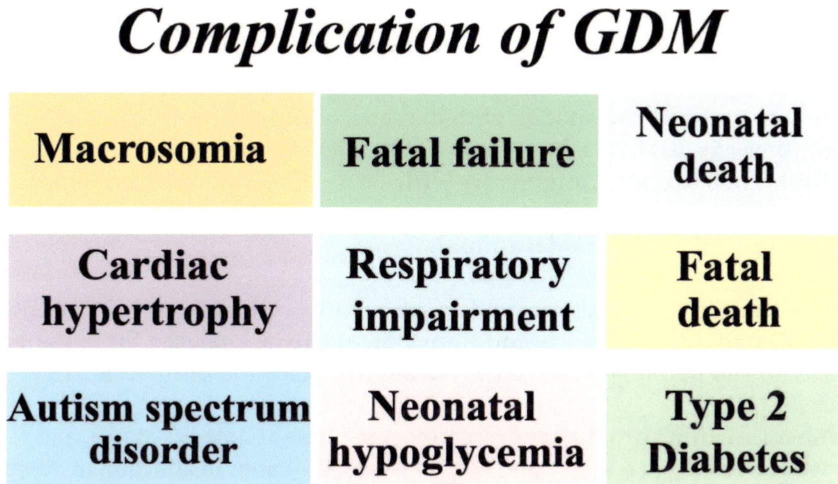

Figure 4.
The neonatal complications of GDM include foetal death, macrosomia, neonatal hypoglycaemia, hyperbilirubinemia, and neonatal respiratory distress syndrome; GDM also puts the mother at increased risk of developing type 2 diabetes (T2D) and cardiovascular disease in the future.

3. Animal model for gestational diabetes mellitus

Diabetes in pregnancy increases the risk of various complications for both the mother and the child. However, the pathogenesis of GDM and its molecular mechanisms have not yet been fully elucidated. Animal and cell models are mainly used in basic research regarding GDM. GDM animal models play a major role in elucidating the pathogenesis and pathophysiology of diabetes, as well as elucidating the mechanisms of its complications. They also provide the theoretical basis for early detection and prevention of GDM and the subsequent clinical dosing and drug evaluation. Diabetes mellitus in humans is associated with complications such as peripheral neuropathy, nephropathy, and retinopathy in about 50% of cases, but there are few animal models that develop all complications; moreover, the animal models are selected according to the research purpose. The most widely used species for diabetes animal models are the mouse and rat. The animal models for type 1 diabetes range from animals that spontaneously develop autoimmune diabetes to those that chemically destroy pancreatic beta cells.

3.1 Spontaneous diabetic models

Spontaneous diabetic animals are not only produced by natural or selective breeding, but also by introducing genes from wild mice. The non-obese diabetic (NOD) mouse and bio breeding (BB) rat are the two most commonly used animals that spontaneously develop diseases similar to human type 1 diabetes. The NOD mouse was established by Makino et al. in the Shionogi Laboratory [30]. The BB rat was discovered in a commercial colony of Wistar-derived rats at the Bio-Breeding Laboratories in Ottawa, Canada [31].

The Goto-Kakizaki (GK) rat was established by Goto and Kakizaki as a non-obese, hypoinsulinemic model of type 2 diabetes [32]. GK rats are a diabetes model mainly due to their trait of non-obesity insulin deficiency established as in an inbred line by selective mating from Wistar rats using impaired glucose tolerance [33]. The Spontaneously Diabetic Torii (SDT) rats were established through inbreeding by selecting and mating Sprague–Dawley rats who developed diabetes [34]. The SDT rat is a novel model of type 2 diabetes that is non-obese, has hypoinsulinemic diabetes, and is characterised by the presence of diabetic retinopathy in individuals with prolonged hyperglycaemia [35]. Diabetes is prominent in males of this model, with diabetes occurring in almost 100% of males at 40 weeks. SDT rats develop proliferative retinopathy and are used as a model for human diabetic retinopathy [36].

3.2 Obese type 2 diabetes model animals

Spontaneous obesity-diabetes models (ob/ob mice, OLETF rat, KK and KKA mice, TSOD mice, SMXA5 mice, and Kuma mice) can be analysed for physiological, biochemical, and pathological changes during the onset and progression of type 2 diabetes [37].

Ob/ob mice exhibit prominent overeating, are obese at 2 weeks of age, and reach a body weight of 40 g at 6 weeks and 60 g at 14 weeks. Later, in addition to overeating and obesity, the mice exhibit hyperglycaemia, hyperinsulinemia, and high blood glucagon levels. Insulin resistance is observed in the peripheral tissues and the liver.

Otsuka Long-Evans Tokushima Fatty (OLETF) rats were established as inbreeding strains through the selective mating of diabetes-developing individuals found in Long-Evans rats. Binge eating obesity is exhibited immediately after weaning, and urinary sugar appears from 40 weeks after birth. Diabetes onset is prominent in males [38].

The KK mouse was established as an inbreeding strain from the experimental mouse produced in the Kasukabe region of the Saitama prefecture in Japan and was named KK mouse after Kasukabe [39]. KK mice are dominated by many diabetic genes, but their pathology is mild. Therefore, the KK-Ay mice were created, wherein the naturally mutated obesity gene, *Ay,* was introduced [40].

KK-Ay mice develop severe obesity and hyperglycaemia 7–8 weeks earlier than KK mice. The incidence of diabetes in males is approximately 100%. Nagoya-Shibata-Yoshida (NSY) mice were established as inbreeding strains by selecting and mating ICR mice with impaired glucose tolerance. Impaired glucose tolerance and elevated blood glucose are exhibited after 8 weeks, and impaired glucose tolerance occurs in almost 100% of males at 48 weeks [41].

Tsumura Suzuki Obese Diabetes (TSOD) mice were established as inbreeding strains by selecting and mating ddY mice, which are highly reproductive non-inbred mice, exhibiting urinary sugar and obesity. During the growth period of 4 to 20 weeks of age, strong overeating is observed, and obesity is exhibited; moreover, hyperglycaemia and abnormal lipid metabolism due to insulin resistance are likewise exhibited. The symptoms are strongly expressed in males [42].

SMXA5 mice are SMXA mice with recombinant inbreeding strains, as well as a high-fat diet-induced type 2 diabetes and fatty liver [43]. Impaired glucose tolerance and hyperinsulinemia frequently develop from 10 weeks of age. For Kuma mice, genome editing technology was used to obtain mice lacking glutamine, the 104th amino acid of the insulin 2 protein, from the immunodeficiency model BRJ mice [44]. This mouse has elevated blood glucose levels after 4 weeks of age.

3.3 Animal model of chemistry-induced diabetes mellitus

Type 1 and type 2 diabetes models can be created by destroying islet of Langerhans cells in the pancreas through drug administration. The main advantages of this method are its relative ease in inducing a model of diabetes, not requiring the use of a specific strain, and the short development time. Most of these animals have type 1 diabetes, but depending on how the drugs are administered, models similar to type 2 diabetes can also be created. The drugs used are streptozotocin (STZ) or alloxan (Alx). STZ is a nitrosourea derivative isolated from *Streptomyces achromogenes* [45]. Drug-induced diabetic rats can also be created from mature rats by intravenous administration of 30 mg/kg STZ or 40 mg/kg Alx. STZ administration to adult rats will produce a type 1 diabetic model, and administration to neonates will produce a type 2 diabetic-like model. Induction is usually done in early pregnancy, before the foetal pancreas has developed, to avoid foetal beta cell destruction by the chemicals being utilised. Alx can create a diabetes model by generating reactive oxygen species (ROS) in the beta cells of the pancreas and destroying these cells.

3.4 Surgically-induced models

Surgical models of diabetes were first created through canine pancreatectomy. In particular, GDM models were created through canine pancreatectomy at various stages of gestation [46]. The disadvantage of this model is that it lacks specificity, as both endocrine and exocrine tissues are removed, causing other symptoms not associated with diabetes mellitus. This is a model of GDM due to insulin deficiency, and not insulin resistance [46]. As mentioned above, there are spontaneous animal models and transgenic animal models of diabetes, but most of them often show remarkable symptoms in males. Since the pregnancy and childbirth of hyperglycaemic mothers are often difficult, the effects of the intrauterine hyperglycaemic environment on children cannot be observed. Thus, we used chemical virulence factors to cause specific damage to the beta cells in the pregnant animal's pancreas, inducing complications similar to GDM. Therefore, we obtained the offspring from the GDM animal model by mating normal Wistar rats and then administering STZ to the tail vein, rather than using diabetic model rats.

4. Intrauterine hyperglycaemia-mimicking cell model

In the case of GDM, foetation is exposed to maternal hyperglycaemia through the placenta during the foetal period. The DOHaD study described in the Introduction mainly focused on the effects of inadequate nutrition during the foetal period (intrauterine undernutrition environment) on the future development of disease in the offspring [4–6]. When the womb provides over-nutrition, the offspring will exhibit numerous complications, as previously described. Recently, studies have been conducted that mimic the hyperglycaemic environment by changing the glucose concentration in the medium using primary cultured cells and cell lines. Nerve cells and skeletal muscle cells, among others, in which cells differentiate and their fate is determined during the foetal period, are important. Although it is possible to use primary cultured cells isolated from foetal organs for these studies, the experiments may be limited because the differentiated cells do not proliferate. Therefore, by using a cell line, the cells can be handled more easily than primary cells.

Myocardial blasts established from rats are often used as heart model cells [47]. The exposure of H9C2 cells to Dulbecco's modified Eagle's medium containing 50 mM high glucose was compared with a medium containing 5.5 mM glucose (the normoglycemic level), and the H9C2 cells reportedly exhibited apoptosis in the high glucose medium [48]. Another study with H9C2 cells showed that simvastatin has an autophagy-mediated cardioprotective effect; this study used a cell model wherein exposure to 200 mM high glucose induced cardiomyocyte apoptosis [49]. Studies using these myocardial blast cell lines suggest that high glucose in an intrauterine hyperglycaemic environment has a profound effect on foetal myocardial blast signalling and proliferation.

PC12 cells, which are pheochromocytoma cells derived from the adrenal gland of *Rattus norvegicus*, are often used in the study of nerve cells [50]. PC12 cells can be differentiated using the nerve growth factor (NGF) to investigate the effects on neurons [51]. Furthermore, high glucose has been shown to cause oxidative stress-induced apoptosis in dopaminergic neurons. Studies with PC-12 cells revealed a correlation between hyperglycaemia and neurodegeneration using a PC-12 cell model exposed in a high glucose medium. Resveratrol, a polyphenol contained in red wine, suppresses nerve cell death due to apoptosis induced by a high glucose environment [52]. Similar studies have been conducted on PC12 cells, indicating that resveratrol or alpha-lipoic acid protected PC12 cells from HG-induced oxidative stress and apoptosis through activation of the PI3K/Akt/FoxO3a signalling pathway [53, 54]. These results suggest that the intrauterine hyperglycaemic environment during pregnancy may lead to inflammation and apoptosis of foetal neurons due to long-term exposure to foetal hyperglycaemia.

Next, we present a study of the effects of high glucose on cells in a skeletal muscle cell model of GDM. Skeletal muscle is an essential organ for energy metabolism. During foetal development, myoblasts differentiate into skeletal muscle during development. Several cell-level studies on how the hyperglycaemic environment affects the differentiation of myoblasts into skeletal muscle are being conducted. In a cell model using mouse myoblasts C2C12, high glucose exposure of 25 mM was shown to accelerate myogenesis by rearranging SUMO enzyme transcripts and SUMO proteins [55]. However, other experiments with C2C12 have shown that even higher glucose concentrations of 60 mM inhibit the expression of the MyoD and myogenin genes, as well as the Akt signal, suppressing skeletal muscle differentiation [56]. High glucose was also shown to interfere with the proliferation of muscle-specific stem cells and satellite cells under adherent culture conditions [57]. Therefore, it is suggested that hyperglycaemia may promote sarcopenia. Glucose is also suggested to be a factor that determines the cell fate of skeletal muscle-specific stem cells. Recently, we found that high glucose (25 mM) in the medium increases the expression of skeletal muscle differentiation marker genes such as MyoD and myogenin compared to normal glucose levels (5 mM), resulting in ROS development and Akt signalling. The differentiation of myoblasts into skeletal muscle was reportedly promoted by high glucose [55]. The appearance of unusually large babies with gestational diabetes complications may be due in part to excessive muscle differentiation.

5. Our study on intrauterine hyperglycaemia

While there have been many studies using animal and cellular models of GDM, few studies have analysed the effects of GDM on the pups born from it. We have previously studied the effects of STZ-induced GDM on the heart of pups using a rat model of GDM. In this section, we describe (1) the effects of a high-fat diet during pregnancy on the hearts of GDM rat pups, (2) the effects of fish oil intake during pregnancy on the hearts of GDM rat pups, and (3) the effects of eicosapentaenoic acid (EPA) intake during pregnancy on primary cardiomyocyte cultures isolated from GDM rat pups.

5.1 Effect of a high-fat diet on stillbirth rate during pregnancy in GDM model rats

GDM model rats were created by administering STZ (50 mg/kg) into the tail vein of Wistar rats on the second day of pregnancy. To investigate the effect of a high-fat diet during pregnancy on the pups, GDM rats were fed a high-fat lard diet (56.7% fat) containing saturated fatty acids and a control diet (7% fat). The stillbirth rate of GDM rats on the high-fat lard diet was much higher than that of GDM on the control diet [58]. Palmitic acid, a saturated fatty acid, has been reported to cause inflammation and cardiac dysfunction in animal and cellular level experiments [59]. In addition to exposure to hyperglycaemia in utero, the consumption of a high-fat lard diet high in saturated fatty acids may have impaired cardiac function in the pups.

5.2 Effect of fish oil intake on the heart of rat pups in the GDM model

In this study, we examined the effects of fish oil (which is rich in ω3 unsaturated fatty acids) on pups, based on reports that fish oil has a positive effect on cardiovascular diseases [60, 61]. GDM rats were fed a high-fat fish oil diet (14% fish oil + 7% lard), a high-fat lard diet rich in saturated fatty acids (21% lard), and a normal diet (7% lard), and the heart signals of the pups were then analysed. The pups of GDM rats fed the lard diet had higher stillbirth rates and triglyceride levels, but these were improved in the pups fed the fish oil diet [62]. An examination of Akt-related signalling revealed that pups born to GDM rats fed a lard diet had reduced levels of Akt phosphorylation, which is important for sugar uptake. Interestingly, however, these signalling abnormalities were ameliorated in the hearts of pups born to GDM rats fed a fish oil diet during pregnancy.

5.3 Effect of EPA intake on primary cardiomyocytes of rat pups in the GDM rat model

Our results indicate that intrauterine hyperglycaemia induces abnormal insulin signalling in the foetal heart. Why does abnormal heart signalling occur

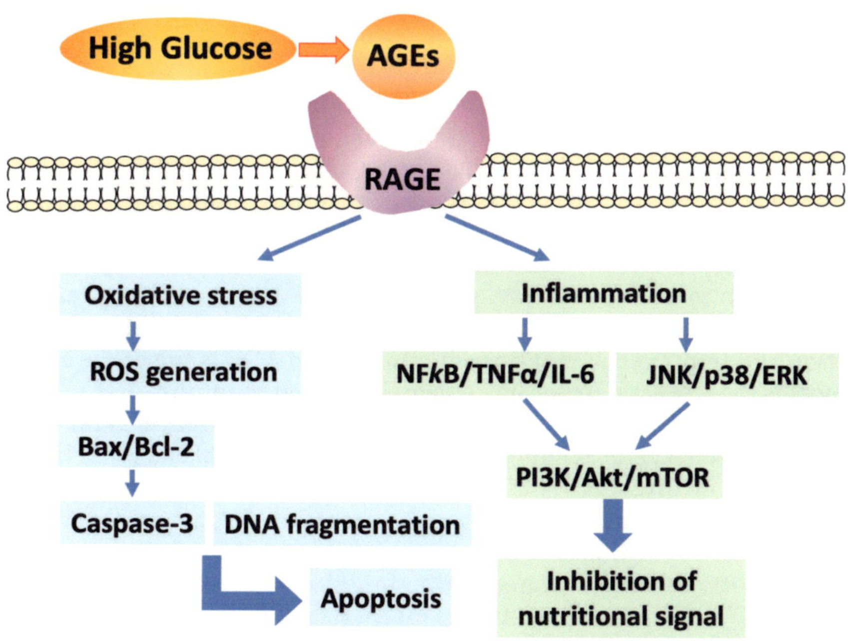

Figure 5.
Prolonged hyperglycaemia leads to excessive glycation of proteins and accumulation of advanced glycation end products (AGEs), which induce inflammation and inhibition of Akt-related signalling, resulting in insulin resistance. In addition, AGEs induced by hyperglycaemia lead to the production of ROS, which in turn induce apoptosis by increasing BAX and degrading caspase.

in the pups? What components of fish oil can be ingested by pregnant mothers to improve the condition? Fish oil is a rich source of the n-3 unsaturated fatty acids EPA and DHA. EPA was chosen as a candidate because it has cardiovascular protective properties, and DHA is biosynthesised by the body from EPA. GDM rats were orally administered EPA through gavage during pregnancy. Primary cardiomyocyte cultures isolated from the hearts of the pups were examined for effects on the insulin signalling system [63]. We found that the inhibition of insulin signalling in primary cardiomyocyte cultures from GDM rats inhibited the translocation of GLUT4 to the plasma membrane. Why do these signalling abnormalities occur? In cultured primary cardiomyocytes from GDM rats, ROS was generated and an increase in excessive protein advanced glycation end products (AGEs) was observed. This AGEsation has been highlighted as a cause of ageing and disease. The accumulation of AGEsed proteins also increases the expression of the receptor of AGEs (RAGE), which triggers AGEs-RAGE signalling. This AGEs-RAGE signalling was found to increase various pro-inflammatory cytokine genes (IL-6, TNFα, and NF-κB) through JNK phosphorylation (**Figure 5**). These results indicate that exposure to hyperglycaemia in the foetus of GDM rats leads to increased AGEs oxidation and chronic inflammation. However, GDM rats fed EPA (an ω3 unsaturated fatty acid) during pregnancy were shown to ameliorate the abnormalities in the pups.

6. Diet and drug therapy for GDM

What other drugs are effective against GDM besides insulin? The effect of using metformin and insulin on GDM has already been reported [64]. Metformin is associated with a decreased incidence of GDM [65]. The weight of metformin-treated neonates is lower than that of insulin-treated neonates. In addition, metformin-treated infants had lower rates of weight gain and malformations during pregnancy than insulin-treated infants. In contrast, metformin-treated infants had greater weight gain in the neonatal period, with no difference in weight between those administered with insulin and metformin. This suggests that weight gain during this period may be linked to cardiovascular disease and indicates the need for additional research. We have previously investigated dietary treatment in GDM rats. EPA, an n-3 unsaturated fatty acid, was administered to GDM rats from day 1 to day 22 of gestation and the effect on new-born rats was investigated. In the heart of puppies born to GDM rats, excessive AGE formation of cardiac proteins impaired signal transduction, but feeding EPA to GDM rats inhibited AGE formation and improved signal transduction. Since AGE is the cause of various diseases [65], several drugs have been developed to inhibit AGEs. The accumulation of AGEs has been reported to induce inflammation and damage vascular endothelial cells, smooth muscle cells, and fibroblasts [66]. In addition to diabetes mellitus, other diseases wherein AGEs are involved include neurodegenerative diseases, cardiovascular diseases, chronic renal failure, and autoimmune diseases [67]. AGE formation inhibitors, AGE destroyers, AGEs-RAGE inhibitors, and signal transduction inhibitors have been previously reported [68–72]. For example, studies on AGE formation inhibitors found that some amino acids in the plasma inhibit glycation by competitively inhibiting the molecular binding of glucose to proteins [73]. Furthermore, AGE-RAGE inhibitors have been shown through animal studies to be protective against diabetic nephropathy when DPP4 is deficient or when DPP4 inhibitors are added [74].

7. Conclusion

Undernutrition or overnutrition during pregnancy has profound effects not only on the mother but also on the child. Children with GDM are focused on neonatal complications, but in the future, they may suffer from lifestyle-related and mental illnesses. Elucidation of these molecular mechanisms is becoming clear using animal models and cell models. Thus, GDM has a major impact on the mother as well as on the child and should be treated rigorously with medication and diet. Insulin is the main drug therapy for controlling blood glucose, but in addition to insulin, insulin resistance improving drugs such as metformin have been tried, but the safety is still unknown. Therefore, dietary management is essential for GDM in addition to safe medication.

Acknowledgements

We gratefully acknowledge the work of past and present members of our laboratory. This work was supported in part by the JSPS KAKENHI Grants (nos. 20 K11611, 15 K00809, and 18 K11136 to AN and RK), the Dairy Products Health Science Council and Japan Dairy Association (to AN), and the Research Program of Jissen Women's University (to AN).

Conflict of interest

The authors declare no conflict of interest.

Author details

Ritsuko Kawaharada[1] and Akio Nakamura[2]*

1 Department of Health and Nutrition, Takasaki University of Health and Welfare, Takasaki, Gunma, Japan

2 Department of Molecular Nutrition, Faculty of Human Life Sciences, Jissen Women's University, Hino, Tokyo, Japan

*Address all correspondence to: nakamura-akio@jissen.ac.jp

References

[1] Barker DJ, Osmond C. Infant mortality, childhood nutrition, and ischaemic heart disease in England and Wales. Lancet .1986;1:1077-1081. doi: 10.1016/s0140-6736(86)91340-1.

[2] Barker DJ. The fetal and infant origins of adult disease. British Medical Journal. 1990;30:1111. doi: 10.1136/bmj.301.6761.1111.

[3] Barker DJ. The origins of the developmental origins theory. Journal of Internal Medicine. 2007;261:412-417. doi: 10.1111/j.1365-2796.2007.01809.x.

[4] Barker DJ, Gluckman, PD,Godfrey KM, et al. Fetal nutrition and cardiovascular disease in adult life. Lancet. 1993;341:938-941. doi: 10.1016/0140-6736(93)91224-a.

[5] Gluckman PD, Hanson MA. Living with the past:evolution, development, and patterns of disease. Science. 2004; 305:1733-1736. doi: 10.1126/science.1095292.

[6] Gluckman PD, Hanson MA:Developmental origins of disease paradigm:a mechanistic and evolutionary perspective. Pediatric research.2004;56:311-317. doi: 10.1203/01.PDR.0000135998.08025.FB.

[7] Roseboom T, Rooij Sd, Painter R. The Dutch famine and its long—term consequences for adult health. Early Human Development.2006;82:485-491. doi: 10.1016/j.earlhumdev.2006.07.001.

[8] Wu L, Feng X, He A, et al.Prenatal exposure to the Great Chinese Famine and mid—age hypertension. PLoS One. 2017;12:e0176413. doi: 10.1371/journal.pone.0176413.

[9] Barker DJ, Osmond C, Forsén TJ, et al. Trajectories of growth among children who have coronary events as adults. The New England Journal of Medicine. 2005;353:1802-1809. doi: 10.1056/NEJMoa044160.

[10] Eriksson JG, Osmond C, Kajantie E, et al. Patterns of growth among children who later develop type 2 diabetes or its risk factors. Diabetologia. 2006;49:2853-2858. doi: 10.1007/s00125-006-0459-1.

[11] Osmond C, Kajantie E, Forsén TJ, et al. Infant growth and stroke in adult life: the Helsinki Birth Cohort Study. Stroke. 2007;38:264-270. doi: 10.1161/01.STR.0000254471.72186.03.

[12] Ylihärsilä H, Kajantie E, Osmond C, et al. Body mass index during childhood and adult body composition in men and women aged 56-70 y. The American Journal of Clinical Nutrition. 2008;87:1769-1775. doi: 10.1093/ajcn/87.6.1769.

[13] International Diabetes Federation: IDF. IDF DIABETES ATLAS 9th edition 2019, https://diabetesatlas.org/en/ [Accessed: 2021-08-01]

[14] Reece EA. Diabetes-induced birth defects: What do we know? What can we do? Current Diabetes Reports. 2012; 12: doi: 10.1007/s11892-011-0251-6.

[15] Reece EA. Perspectives on obesity, pregnancy and birth outcomes in the United States: The scope of the problem. American Journal of Obstetrics & Gynecolog. 2008;198: 23-27. doi: 10.1016/j.ajog.2007.06.076.

[16] Reece EA. The fetal and maternal consequences of gestational diabetes mellitus. The Journal of Maternal-Fetal & Neonatal Medicine. 2010; 23: 199-203. doi: 10.3109/14767050903550659.

[17] Feig DS, Palda VA. Type 2 diabetes in pregnancy: A growing concern. Lancet 2002; 359: 1690-1692.doi: 10.1016/S0140-6736(02)08599-9.

[18] Harris BS, Bishop KC, Kemeny HR, et al. Risk Factors for Birth Defects. Obstetrical & Gynecological Survey. 2017; 72: 123-135. doi: 10.1097/OGX.0000000000000405.

[19] Schneider S, Bock C, Wetzel M, et al. The prevalence of gestational diabetes in advanced economies. Journal of Perinatal Medicine. 2012; 40, 511-520. doi: 10.1515/jpm-2012-0015.

[20] Kong L, Nilsson IAK, Gissler M, et al. Associations of Maternal Diabetes and Body Mass Index with Offspring Birth Weight and Prematurity. JAMA Pediatrics. 2019; 173: 371-378. doi: 10.1001/jamapediatrics.2018.5541.

[21] ACOG: Practice Bulletin No: 190: gestational diabetes mellitus. Obstetrics & Gynecology. 2018;131:e49–e64. doi: 10.1097/AOG.0000000000002501.

[22] Chiefari E, Arcidiacono B, Foti D, et al. Gestational diabetes mellitus: an updated overview. Journal of Endocrinological Investigation. 2017; 40:899-909. doi: 10.1007/s40618-016-0607-5.

[23] Schneider S, Bock C, Wetzel M, et al. The prevalence of gestational diabetes in advanced economies. Journal of Perinatal Medicine. 2012;40:511-520.

[24] Kong L, Nilsson IAK, Gissler M, et al. Associations of Maternal Diabetes and Body Mass Index with Offspring Birth Weight and Prematurity. JAMA Pediatrics. 2019;173:371-378. doi: 10.1001/jamapediatrics.2018.5541.

[25] Metzger BE, Lowe LP, Dyer AR, et al. Hyperglycemia and adverse pregnancy outcomes. The New England Journal of Medicine. 2008;358:1991-2002.

[26] Metzger BE, Gabbe SG, Persson B, et al. International association of diabetes and pregnancy study groups recommendations on the diagnosis and classification of hyperglycemia in pregnancy. Diabetes Care. 2010;33:676-682. doi: 10.2337/dc09-1848.

[27] HAPO Study Cooperative Research Group, Metzger BE, Lowe LP, et al. Hyperglycemia and adverse pregnancy outcomes. The New England Journal of Medicine. 2008;358:1991-2002. doi: 10.1056/NEJMoa0707943.

[28] Clausen TD, Mathiesen ER, Hansen T, et al. High prevalence of type 2 diabetes and pre-diabetes in adult offspring of women with gestational diabetes mellitus or type 1 diabetes: the role of intrauterine hyperglycemia. Diabetes Care. 2008;31:340-346. doi: 10.2337/dc07-1596.

[29] Sugihara S, Sasaki N, Amemiya S, et al. Analysis of weight at birth and at diagnosis of childhood-onset type 2 diabetes mellitus in Japan. Pediatric Diabetes. 2008;9:285-290. doi: 10.1111/j.1399-5448.

[30] Makino S, Kunimoto K, Munaoko Y, et al. Breeding of a non-obese diabetic strain of mice. Jikken Dobutsu.1980; 29: 1-13. doi: 10.1538/expanim1978.29.1_1.

[31] Nakhooda AF, Like AA, Chappel CI, et al. The spontaneously diabetic wistar rat. Metabolic and morphological studies. Diabetes 1977; 26:100-112. doi: 10.2337/diab.26.2.100.

[32] Goto Y, Kakizaki M, Masaki N. Spontaneous diabetes produced by selective breeding of normal Wistar rats. Proceedings of the Japan Academy.1975; 51:80-85.

[33] Goto Y, Kakizaki M, Masaki N. Production of spontaneous diabetic rats by repetition of selective breeding. The Tohoku Journal of Experimental Medicine. 1976;119: 85-90. doi: 10.1620/tjem.119.85.

[34] Shinohara M, Masuyama T, Shoda T, et al. A new spontaneously diabetic

non-obese Torii rat strain with severe ocular complications. International journal of experimental diabetes research. 2000; 1(2): 89-100. doi: 10.1155/edr.2000.89.

[35] Coleman DL, Hummel KP. The influence of genetic background on the expression of the obese (ob) gene in the mouse. Diabetologia. 1973;9:287-293. doi: 10.1155/edr.2000.89

[36] Kawano K, Hirashima T, Mori S, et al. Spontaneous long-term hyperglycemic rat with diabetic complications Otsuka Long-Evans Tokushima Fatty (OLETF) strain. Diabetes. 1992;41:1422-1428. doi: 10.2337/diab.41.11.1422.

[37] Nakamura M, Yamada K. Studies on a diabetic (KK) strain of the mouse. Diabetologia. 1967;3(2):212-221. doi: 10.1007/BF01222198.

[38] Nishimura M. Breeding of mice strains for diabetes mellitus. Experimental Animals. 1969; 18: 147-147.

[39] Shibata M, Yasuda B. New experimental congenital diabetic mice (N.S.Y. mice). The Tohoku Journal of Experimental Medicine. 1980;130:139-142. doi: 10.1620/tjem.130.139.

[40] Tabuchi M, Funo S, Yanagisawa T, et al. A new mouse model of spontaneous diabetes derived from ddY strain. Suzuki W, Iizuka S, Experimental Animals. 1999;48:181-189. doi: 10.1538/expanim.48.181.

[41] Kobayashi M, Ohno T, Tsuji A, et al. Combinations of nondiabetic parental genomes elicit impaired glucose tolerance in mouse SMXA recombinant inbred strains. Diabetes. 2003;52: 180-186. doi: 10.2337/diabetes.52.1.180.

[42] Sakano D, Inoue A, Enomoto T, et al. Insulin2Q104del (Kuma) mutant mice develop diabetes with dominant inheritance. Scientific Reports. 2020;10:12187. doi: 10.1038/s41598-020-68987-z.

[43] Bono VH. Review of mechanism of action studies of the nitrosureas. Cancer treatment reports. 1976; 60: 699-702.

[44] Rerup CC. Drugs producing diabetes through damage of the insulin secreting cells. Pharmacological Reviews. 1970;22:485-518.

[45] Lenzen S, Patten U. Alloxan: history and mechanism of action. Diabetologia. 1988;31:337- 342. doi: 10.1007/BF02341500.

[46] Pasek RC, Gannon M. Advancements and challenges in generating accurate animal models of gestational diabetes mellitus. Vol. 305, American Journal of Physiology-Endocrinology and Metabolism. 2013; 305:E1327-1338. doi: 10.1152/ajpendo.00425.2013.

[47] Kimes BW, Brandt BL. Properties of a clonal muscle cell line from rat heart. Exp. Cell Res. 1976;98: 367-381. doi: 10.1016/0014-4827(76)90447-x.

[48] Han s, Wang G, Jin Y, et al. Investigating the Mechanism of Hyperglycemia-Induced Fetal Cardiac Hypertrophy. PLoS One. 2015; 29;10:e0139141. DOI: 10.1371/journal.pone.0139141

[49] Lusha E and Hong J. Simvastatin protects high glucose-induced H9c2 cells from injury by inducing autophagy. Pharm Biol. 2020; 58: 1077-1084. doi: 10.1371/journal.pone.0139141.

[50] Weber E, Jilling T, Kirk KL. Distinct functional properties of Rab3A and Rab3B in PC12 neuroendocrine cells. Journal of Biological Chemistry. 1996;271:6963-6971. doi: 10.1074/jbc.271.12.6963.

[51] Renaud J, Bournival J, Zottig X, et al. Resveratrol Protects DAergic PC12

Cells from High Glucose-Induced Oxidative Stress and Apoptosis: Effect on p53 and GRP75 Localization, Neurotoxicity Research. 2014;25:110-123. doi: 10.1007/s12640-013-9439-7

[52] Liu MH, Yuan C, He J, et al. Resveratrol protects PC12 cells from high glucose-induced neurotoxicity via PI3K/Akt/FoxO3a pathway. Cellular and Molecular Neurobiology. 2015;35:513-522. doi: 10.1007/s10571-014-0147-5.

[53] Yan T, Zhang Z, Li D. NGF receptors and PI3K/AKT pathway involved in glucose fluctuation-induced damage to neurons and alpha-lipoic acid treatment. BMC Neuroscience. 2020;21:38. doi: 10.1186/s12868-020-00588-y.

[54] Liu X, Heras G, Lauschke VM, et al. High glucose-induced oxidative stress accelerates myogenesis by altering SUMO reactions. Experimental Cell Research. 2020;395:112234. doi: 10.1016/j.yexcr.2020.112234.

[55] Luo W, Ai L, Wang BF, et al. High glucose inhibits myogenesis and induces insulin resistance by down-regulating AKT signaling. Biomedicine & Pharmacotherapy. 2019;120:109498. doi: 10.1016/j.biopha.2019.109498.

[56] Furuichi Y, Kawabata Y, Aoki M, et al. Excess Glucose Impedes the Proliferation of Skeletal Muscle Satellite Cells Under Adherent Culture Conditions. Frontiers in Cell and Developmental Biology. 2021;9:640399. doi: 10.3389/fcell.2021.640399.

[57] Tokunaga Y, Yoshizaki H, Toriumi A, et al. Effects of omega-7 palmitoleic acids on skeletal muscle differentiation in a hyperglycemic condition. The Journal of Veterinary Medical Science. 2021. doi: 10.1292/jvms.21-0309.

[58] Nasu R, Seki K, Nara M, et al. Effect of a high-fat diet on diabetic mother rats and their offspring through three generations. Endocrine Journal. 2007; 54: 563-569. doi: 10.1507/endocrj.k06-175.

[59] Hooper L, Martin N, Abdelhamid A, Reduction in saturated fat intake for cardiovascular disease. Cochrane Database of Systematic Reviews, 2015;6: CD011737. doi: 10.1002/14651858.CD011737.

[60] Park S, Park Y. Effects of dietary fish-oil and trans fat on rat aorta histopathology and cardiovascular risk markers. Nutrition Research and Practice. 2009;3:102-107. doi: 10.4162/nrp.2009.3.2.102.

[61] Kromhout D, Geleijnse JM, de Goede J, et al. n-3 fatty acids, ventricular arrhythmia-related events, and fatal myocardial infarction in postmyocardial infarction patients with diabetes. Diabetes Care. 2011; 34:2515-2520. DOI: 10.2337/dc11-0896

[62] Nasu-Kawaharada R, Nakamura A, Kakarla S, et al. A maternal diet rich in fish oil may improve cardiac Akt-related signaling in the offspring of diabetic mother rats. Nutrition. 2013;29; 688-692. doi: 10.1016/j.nut.2012.11.017.

[63] Kawaharada R, Masuda H, Chen Z, et al. Intrauterine hyperglycemia-induced inflammatory signalling via the receptor for advanced glycation end products in the cardiac muscle of the infants of diabetic mother rats. European Journal of Nutrition. 2018;57:2701-2712. doi: 10.1007/s00394-017-1536-6.

[64] Tarry-AdkinsID JL, Aiken CE, Ozanne SE. Neonatal, infant, and childhood growth following metformin versus insulin treatment for gestational diabetes: A systematic review and meta-analysis. PLOS Medicine. 2019;16: e1002848. doi: .1371/journal.pmed.1002848.

[65] Priya G, Kalra S. Drugs Context. Metformin in the management of diabetes during pregnancy and lactation. 2018; 7: 212523. doi: 10.7573/dic.212523.

[66] Kawaharada R, Masuda H, Chen Z, et al. Intrauterine hyperglycemia-induced inflammatory signalling via the receptor for advanced glycation end products in the cardiac muscle of the infants of diabetic mother rats. Eur J Nutr. 2018; 57: 2701-2712. doi: 10.1007/s00394-017-1536-6.

[67] Shen C-Y, Lu C-H, Wu C-H , et al. The Development of Maillard Reaction, and Advanced Glycation End Product (AGE)-Receptor for AGE (RAGE) Signaling Inhibitors as Novel Therapeutic Strategies for Patients with AGE-Related Diseases. Molecules. 2020; 25: 5591. doi: 10.3390/molecules25235591.

[68] Reddy VP, Beyaz A. Inhibitors of the Maillard reaction and AGE breakers as therapeutics for multiple diseases. Drug Discovery Today. 2006; 11: 646-654. doi: 10.1016/j.drudis.2006.05.016.

[69] Sourris KC, Harcourt BE, Forbes JM. A new perspective on therapeutic inhibition of advanced glycation in diabetic microvascular complications: Common downstream endpoints achieved through disparate therapeutic approaches? American Journal of Nephrology. 2009; 30: 323-335. doi: 10.1159/000226586.

[70] Younus H, Anwar S. Prevention of non-enzymatic glycosylation (glycation): Implication in the treatment of diabetic complication. International Journal of Health Sciences. 2016; 10: 261-277.

[71] Abbas G, Al-Harrasi AS, Hussain H, et al. Antiglycation therapy:Discovery of promising antiglycation agents for the management of diabetic complications. Pharm. Biol. 2016, 54, 198-206. doi: 10.3109/13880209.2015.1028080.

[72] Rowan S, Bejarano E, Taylor A. Mechanistic targeting of advanced glycation end-products in age-related diseases. Biochimica et Biophysica Acta - Molecular Basis of Disease. 2018; 1864: 3631-3643. doi: 10.1016/j.bbadis.2018.08.036.

[73] Chilukuri H, Kulkarni MJ, Fernandes M. Revisiting amino acids and peptides as anti-glycation agents. MedChemComm. 2018; 9: 614-624. doi: 10.1039/c7md00514h.

[74] Yamagishi S, Nakamura N, Suematsu M. et al. Advanced glycation end products:A molecular target for vascular complications in diabetes. Molecular Medicine. 2015; 21, S32–S40. doi: 10.2119/molmed.2015.00067.